NUTRITION AND DIET RESEARCH PROGRESS

MAINTAINING A HEALTHY DIET

NUTRITION AND DIET RESEARCH PROGRESS

Diet Quality of Americans
Nancy Cole and Mary Kay Fox
2009. ISBN: 978-1-60692-777-9
2009. ISBN: 978-1-60876-499-0 (E-book)

School Nutrition and Children
Thomas J. Baxter (Editor)
2009. ISBN: 978-1-60692-891-2

Appetite and Nutritional Assessment
Shane J. Ellsworth
and Reece C. Schuster (Editors)
2009. ISBN: 978-1-60741-085-0

Beta Carotene: Dietary Sources, Cancer and Cognition
Leiv Haugen and Terje Bjornson (Editors)
2009. ISBN: 978-1-60741-611-1

Flavonoids: Biosynthesis, Biological Effects and Dietary Sources
Raymond B. Keller (Editor)
2009. ISBN: 978-1-60741-622-7

Handbook of Vitamin C Research: Daily Requirements, Dietary Sources and Adverse Effects
Hubert Kucharski and Julek Zajac (Editors)
2009. ISBN: 978-1-60741-874-0

Supercritical Fluid Technology Applied to the Manufacture of Prebiotic Carbohydrates
Tiziana Fornari, Fernando Montañés, Agustín Olano and Elena Ibáñez
2010. ISBN: 978-1-60876-978-0

Biological Effects of β -Carotene
Rosa Martha Perez Gutierrez, Adriana Maria Neira Gonzalez and Sandra Lugardo Diaz
2010. ISBN: 978-1-61668-256-9
2010. ISBN: 978-1-61668-609-3 (E-book)

Nutritional Education
Ida R. Laidyth (Editor)
2010. ISBN: 978-1-60876-078-7

Dietary Supplements: Primer and FDA Oversight
Timothy H. Riley (Editor)
2010. ISBN: 978-1-60741-891-7

Handbook of Nutritional Biochemistry: Genomics, Metabolomics and Food Supply
Sondre Haugen and Simen Meijer (Editors)
2010. ISBN: 978-1-60741-916-7

Dietary Fiber, Fruit and Vegetable Consumption and Health
Friedrich Klein and Georg Möller (Editors)
2010. ISBN: 978-1-60876-025-1

Maintaining a Healthy Diet
Anna R. Bernstein (Editor)
2010. ISBN: 978-1-60741-856-6

Nutritional Factors and Osteoporosis Prevention
Masayoshi Yamaguchi
2010. ISBN: 978-1-60876-929-2

Vitamin D: Biochemistry, Nutrition and Roles
William J. Stackhouse (Editor)
2010. ISBN: 978-1-61668-273-6
2010. ISBN: 978-1-61668-713-7 (E-book)

Phytochemicals for the Control of Human Appetite and Body Weight

S.A. Tucci, E.J. Boyland and J.C. Halford

2010. ISBN: 978-1-61668-676-5

2010. ISBN: 978-1-61668-897-4 (E-book)

N-3 Fats: Nutritional Needs, Traditional and Novel Sources| and Microbial Production Strategies

Anita Nordeng Jakobsen

2010. ISBN: 978-1-61668-687-1

2010. ISBN: 978-1-61728-238-6 (E-book)

Green Tea and Beyond

Christine Hurley Deriso and Stephen Hsu

2010. ISBN: 978-1-61668-845-5

2010. ISBN: 978-1-61728-456-4 (E-book)

NUTRITION AND DIET RESEARCH PROGRESS

MAINTAINING A HEALTHY DIET

ANNA R. BERNSTEIN
EDITOR

Nova Science Publishers, Inc.
New York

For permission to use material from this book please contact us:
Telephone 631-231-7269; Fax 631-231-8175
Web Site: http://www.novapublishers.com

LIBRARY OF CONGRESS CATALOGING-IN-PUBLICATION DATA

Maintaining a healthy diet / editor, Anna R. Bernstein.
p. ; cm.
Includes bibliographical references and index.
ISBN 978-1-60741-856-6 (softcover)
1. Nutrition policy--United States. I. Bernstein, Anna R.
[DNLM: 1. Diet--United States--Collected Works. 2. Health Promotion--United States--Collected Works. 3. Feeding Behavior--United States--Collected Works. 4. Health Behavior--United States--Collected Works. 5. Nutrition Policy--United States--Collected Works. 6. Obesity--prevention & control--United States--Collected Works. QT 235 M226 2009]
TX360.U6M35 2009
363.19'262--dc22 2009039012

Published by Nova Science Publishers, Inc. ✝ New York

CONTENTS

PREFACE

This book is a focus on the USDA and other public health agencies that have a long history of disseminating information about why and how to make food choices that promote health and prevent disease. Since 1980, recommendations on attaining adequate nutrition also include information about the benefits of maintaining a healthy body weight and limiting consumption of nutrients linked to chronic diseases. On the other side of the table, food manufacturers and marketers have discovered that certain psychological cues, such as packaging and presentation, are efficient ways to increase consumption of their products. These approaches have not been widely used in public health efforts aimed at improving diet quality and reducing body weight. The sharp increase in overweight and obesity among Americans has occurred concurrently with increased awareness and publicity regarding the benefits of a healthy lifestyle. Examining this phenomenon provides an opportunity to incorporate elements of behavioral economics into consumer food choice analysis.This book consists of public documents which have been located, gathered, combined, reformatted, and enhanced with a subject index, selectively edited and bound to provide easy access.

Chapter 1 - Poor diets and rising obesity rates among Americans have persisted despite increased awareness and publicity regarding the benefits of a healthy lifestyle. This analysis of consumer food choice developed a consumer demand model to illustrate how both long-term health objectives and immediate visceral influences—long intervals between meals and away-from-home eating—can affect individuals' food choices. The model predicts that dietary knowledge will have less influence on food choices in the face of imme-diate visceral factors. The model predictions were tested using data from the 1994-96 Continuing Survey of Food Intake by Individuals and the companion Diet Health and

Knowledge Survey. Longer intervals between meals and consumption of more food away from home both contribute to one's consuming more calories and more calories from solid fats, alcohol, and added sugars. Longer intervals between meals are also associated with lower diet quality.

Chapter 2 - Findings from behavioral and psychological studies indicate that people regularly and predictably behave in ways that contradict some standard assumptions of economic analysis. Recognizing that consumption choices are determined by factors other than prices, income, and information illuminates a broad array of strategies to influence consumers' food choices. These strategies expand the list of possible ideas for improving the diet quality and health of participants in the U.S. Department of Agricul-ture's (USDA) Food Stamp Program; the Special Supplemental Nutrition Program for Women, Infants, and Children (WIC); and the National School Lunch and School Breakfast Programs.

Chapter 3 - This report examines major trends in the amount of food available for consumption in the United States between 1970 and 2005 using data from the ERS Food Availability (Per Capita) Data System. The report also estimates whether Americans are meeting Federal dietary recommendations for each of the major food groups by comparing the data with dietary recommendations in the *2005 Dietary Guidelines for Americans* and the MyPyramid Food Guidance System. Findings show that Americans do not meet the Federal dietary recommendations. In order to meet them, Americans would need to substantially lower their intake of added fats, refined grains, and added sugars and sweeteners and increase their consumption of fruits, vegetables, whole grains, and low-fat milk and milk products.

In: Maintaining a Healthy Diet
Editor: Anna R. Bernstein
ISBN: 978-1-60741-856-6

Chapter 1

IS DIETARY KNOWLEDGE ENOUGH? HUNGER, STRESS, AND OTHER ROADBLOCKS TO HEALTHY EATING

Lisa Mancino and Jean Kinsey

ABSTRACT

Poor diets and rising obesity rates among Americans have persisted despite increased awareness and publicity regarding the benefits of a healthy lifestyle. This analysis of consumer food choice developed a consumer demand model to illustrate how both long-term health objectives and immediate visceral influences—long intervals between meals and away-from-home eating—can affect individuals' food choices. The model predicts that dietary knowledge will have less influence on food choices in the face of imme-diate visceral factors. The model predictions were tested using data from the 1994-96 Continuing Survey of Food Intake by Individuals and the companion Diet Health and Knowledge Survey. Longer intervals between meals and consumption of more food away from home both contribute to one's consuming more calories and more calories from solid fats, alcohol, and added sugars. Longer intervals between meals are also associated with lower diet quality.

Keywords: behavioral economics, food consumption, obesity, fixed effects, instrumental variables.

ACKNOWLEDGMENTS

The authors greatly appreciate the thoughtful review suggestions from Joanne Guthrie, Economic Research Service (ERS); Dianne Whitmore Shazenbach, University of Chicago; Wen You, Virginia Tech; and Carol Olander, Food and Nutrition Service (FNS). We also thank Dale Simms for editorial expertise and Wynnice Pointer-Napper for layout and design.

SUMMARY

Poor diets and rising obesity rates among Americans have occurred concurrently with increased awareness and publicity regarding the benefits of a healthy lifestyle. This seeming contradiction provides an opportunity to incorporate elements of behavioral economics into consumer food choice analysis. This report presents a consumer demand model to illustrate how both long-term health objectives and immediate visceral infl uences—long intervals between meals, eating away from home, or time pressures—can drive individuals' food choices.

What Is the Issue?

A better understanding of how situational factors affect food choices will strengthen public programs aimed at improving diet, health, and nutrition. Knowing when individuals are more likely to forgo health concerns may suggest ways to combat the effect of such situations or to identify commitment mechanisms more in keeping with long-term health goals. And the likely relationship between visceral factors and food choices implies that analysis over shorter time periods, such as per eating occasion, may uncover important information that is hidden when food choices are aggregated over an entire day or more.

What Did the Project Find?

When individuals extend the interval between meals or consume more of their food away from home, they are significantly more likely to consume more calories and more calories from solid fats, alcohol, and added sugars (discretionary calories) at each eating occasion. For example, going 5 hours between meals instead of 4 adds about 52 calories for someone on a diet of 2,000 calories per day; extending that interval from 4 to 6 hours would add about 91 calories to the meal.

Going longer stretches between meals is also estimated to lower diet quality at each meal. The location at which someone makes his or her food choices and when these choices are made significantly affect what and how much is consumed. Not surprisingly, people are estimated to cosume more calo-ries when eating foods from a restaurant compared with foods prepared at home—about 107 more calories per meal.

The model suggests that people who work more hours in a week—a proxy for time pressures—are also more influenced by the interval between meals than those who work fewer hours. As an individual who works more hours in a week goes longer between meals, he or she will choose a meal that is significantly higher in calories, higher in discretionary calories, and lower in diet quality. At 4 hours between meals, an individual who works 40 hours a week is estimated to eat about 20 percent more calories than someone who is not employed. At 8 hours between meals, the calorie discrepancy jumps to nearly 40 percent.

Our model shows that a situational change in caloric intake and diet quality is more pronounced among individuals who are less informed about diet and nutrition. A person with a knowledge score of 50 (from USDA's Diet and Health Knowledge Survey) is estimated to increase per-meal caloric intake by about 28 percent when eating away from home, while a person whose score is 100 points is estimated to eat about only 12 percent more calories.

As people change their dietary goals based on prevailing nutritional beliefs, situational factors like hunger and time pressures will continue to interfere with long-term health objectives. Making specific reference to such situations and suggesting ways to mitigate their effects should enhance the usefulness of educational campaigns designed to improve diet quality. For example, encour-aging consumers to take more active control in limiting the interval between meals and choosing nutrient-dense snacks, such as fruits and vegetables, may help them better align their intentions to eat well with their actual behavior. Limiting intake of foods prepared away from home is also estimated to signifi -cantly decrease caloric consumption. Thus, another possibility would be to encourage individuals to plan ahead or seek out information about nutrient and caloric content of foods prepared away from home.

How Was the Project Conducted?

A theoretical model of both long-term health objectives and short-term situational factors affecting food choices predicts that when individuals face intense visceral influences, such as hunger or stress, their information about health and nutrition will have a smaller impact. It also predicts that individuals who are less informed about health and nutrition, or face higher levels of stress, will be more likely to eschew their long-term goals when faced with visceral factors such as hunger. These hypotheses are tested using data from the 1994-96 Continuing Survey of Food Intake by Individuals and the companion Diet Health and Knowledge Survey, both administered by USDA. The analysis of choices made at each eating occasion enables the use of a fixed-effects estimator. This then controls for the endogeneity between dietary information and food choices. Instrumental variable estima-tors further account for endogeneity that may exist between food choices and meal timing.

INTRODUCTION

The public policy approach to improving the nutritional quality of Americans' diets has relied heavily on disseminating information, such as MyPyramid, about why and how to make food choices that promote health and prevent disease (USDA, 2006). Educational efforts like this may be paying dividends. For example, a 2001 study found that nearly 60 percent of sampled shoppers indicated that their grocery purchases were strongly affected by some health concern and 76 percent felt that healthy eating was a better way to manage their health than medication. These statistics had increased to 80 percent and 86 percent by 2002 (FMI, 2001, 2002). Sales of organic foods increased 17-21 percent per year between 1997 and 2004. Sales of functional/ fortified foods increased 34 percent between 2003 and 2004, whereas total food sales increased 2.4 percent over the same period (Food Institute Reports, 2004, 2005). In addition, the large volume of diet books and products sold to

American consumers suggests we are aware of diet and health issues, curious about slimming down, and mindful of good health (Ackman, 2005).

While shopper surveys and sales figures imply a national interest in improving diet, aggregate health statistics do not reflect these concerns. As of 2003-04, 66 percent of American adults were overweight and over one-third were also obese. Between 1976 and 2000, the number of individuals classi-fied as obese more than doubled (Centers for Disease Control and Prevention (CDC), 2003).[1] During the same time span, there was a parallel rise in the incidence of diseases highly correlated with poor nutrition and overconsumption: cancer, strokes, heart disease, and diabetes (Surgeon General, 2001). In 2000, obesity accounted for an estimated $117 billion a year in direct and indirect economic costs; diabetes is estimated to account for another $132 billion (CDC, 2005).

These conflicting trends highlight a disturbing inconsistency. While Americans demonstrate a concern about eating well and using diet to manage their health, they are getting heavier and increasing their risk of suffering from diet-related illnesses. A rift between long-term objectives and short-term desires can lead to time-inconsistent choices, where people switch their preference for a smaller, yet more immediate, reward over a larger but delayed reward when the time delay between receiving either reward is changed equally. A common example describes an individual who prefers 1 apple right now to 2 apples tomorrow, yet also prefers 2 apples in 51 days to 1 apple in 50 days (Thaler, 1981). Understanding which situations are more conducive to making these seemingly inconsistent choices can improve our understanding of the sometimes tenuous relationship between diet/health knowledge and food choices.

The burgeoning literature on behavioral economics suggests that insights gleaned from economic analysis can be improved by incorporating the presence and level of confounding factors, such as drive states (e.g., hunger, pain, fear), environmental factors, and other short-term circumstances (Loewenstein, 1996, 2000; Laibson, 2001; Read and van Leeuwen, 1998; Herman and Polivy, 2003). In turn, this may clarify how and when inten-tions are more likely to translate to actual behavior. The model developed by Loewenstein (1996) shows that in the presence of intense visceral factors, such as hunger, thirst, or addiction, an individual will be compelled to make choices that undermine long-term health objectives. Using experimental results in conjunction with Loewenstein's model of visceral factors, Read and van Leeuwen (1998) found subjects' levels of hunger to be signifi cantly correlated with observed inconsistencies. The snacks chosen for immediate consumption were significantly less healthful than those chosen for future consumption, while for both future and immediate consumption, the choices made by hungry individuals were less healthful. Herman and Polivy (2003) also examined whether behavioral economics models might be appropriate for the study of dieting and food choice. They find that when presented with tempting foods, dieters are more likely to display uninhibited eating in the presence of some motivational disruptions, such as emotional arousal, intoxication, or distress.

These findings indicate that there are situations where individuals behave in ways contrary to their own long-term self-interests. As O'Donoghue and Rabin (1999) point out, evidence of present-biased preferences brings up complex questions for public policy. In terms of obesity and poor nutrition, time-consistent preferences assume that an overweight or unhealthful individual may be making an optimal choice if he or she derives more pleasure from unhealthy behaviors than good health. As such, a heavy-handed nutrition policy, like taxing unhealthy foods to raise diet quality, would unambiguously make that person worse off. On the other hand, present-biased preferences assume that, while a person may respond rationally to current situations and make unhealthful choices, finding incentives that would make one less responsive to these situations will improve long-term well-being.

Such findings have important implications for econometric analysis of consumers' food choices. For one, empirical estimation that does not include relevant visceral factors, such as an individual's level of hunger, will yield biased estimates of the relationship between dietary information and food choices. Also, a better understanding of how situational factors affect food choices will strengthen programs aimed at improving diet, nutrition, and health outcomes. Knowing when individuals may be more likely to forgo health concerns might suggest ways to reduce the deleterious impact of such situations, or to identify commitment mechanisms that help individuals make choices that are more in keeping with their own long-term health goals.

Another important implication of the likely relationship between visceral factors and food choices is that analysis over shorter time periods, such as per eating occasion, may uncover important information that is hidden when food choices are aggregated over an entire day or more. Using the Continuing Survey of Food Intakes by Individuals (CSFII) and Diet and Health Knowledge Survey (DHKS) data to analyze food choices on this level transforms what is traditionally a cross-sectional data set into one more akin to a panel data set. This provides an opportunity to employ fi xed-effects estimators, and this circumvents some of the endogeneity issues that can plague cross-sectional analysis of food demand. Instrumental variable estimators further reduce problems of endogeneity.

THEORETICAL BACKGROUND

In economics, food can be viewed as both a consumption good and an investment. Through flavor, texture, and relief from hunger, food provides immediate gratification. Through nutrients and calories, it also confers costs and benefits for future health and well-being. Thus, economic models often employ a dynamic framework to model demand for health (Grossman, 1972), nutrient intake (Behrman and Deolalikar, 1990; Barrett, 2002), food choices as they relate to health and labor market activities (Pitt et al., 1990), and food choices as they relate to health and body weight (Cawley, 2004; Cutler et al., 2003). Typically, such models assume that individuals maximize utility over some timeframe using a discounted utility model:

$$U_t(c_t,\ldots,c_T)=U(c_t)+\sum_{\tau=1}^{T}\delta^{\tau}\,U(c_{t+\tau}).$$

In this model, $U(c_{t+\tau})$ is considered to be the individual's well-being at time $t + \tau$, and δ^{τ} is the individual's discount function, or the relative weight attached at time τ to one's well-being in period $t + \tau$. As such, the value we place on future well-being is less than the value of today's well-being, and the value of each subsequent period decreases at a constant rate. Although this assumption—referred to as *exponential discounting*—has become the norm in economic analysis, empirical findings often violate its theoretical predictions or underlying assumptions (Frederick et al., 2003). One frequently observed anomaly is that individuals tend to behave more patiently (by making choices that are consistent with their future savings or health goals) when evaluating tradeoffs that will occur at some point in the future than they would if these same tradeoffs were to occur more immedi-ately. For example, most individuals will prefer \$110 in 31 days over \$100 in 30 days. Yet many of these same individuals will also prefer \$100 right now over \$110 tomorrow. In contrast, an exponential discounting model would predict that an individual who chooses \$110 in 31 days over \$100 in 30 would also choose \$110 tomorrow over \$100 today.

Repeated observance of time-inconsistent preferences has led some researchers to develop models in which individuals have preferences that are biased to prefer immediate rewards and delayed costs. These *present-biased preferences* allow individuals to have a declining discount rate between now and the next period, and a constant discount rate from then on. The result is that individuals will prefer an alternative that is usually less desirable or valuable over some time period simply because it is available sooner. These models have been extended to model individual consumption and savings behavior (Thaler and Shefrin, 1981; Akerlof 1991; Ainslie and Haslam, 1992; Laibson, 1997; Mullainathan and Thaler, 2000; O'Donoghue and Rabin, 1999, 2001).[2] They have also been used to explain why individuals have problems related to self-control, why they demonstrate reversals in preference, and how they can improve their longrun well-being through some commitment, such as 401(k) plans, that limit current consumption levels and thereby preclude procrastination.

For food choice analysis, these models may not be entirely applicable because time-inconsistent behavior is attributed entirely to a reward's temporal proximity (Frederick et al., 2003; Loewenstein, 1996, 2000). In terms of food consumption, this means an individual will always be expected to choose the more immediately available food, regardless of his or her level of hunger. In reviewing the literature on weight loss, Herman and Polivy (2003) emphasize that making food immediately available is not suffi cient to induce uninhibited eating bouts. Loewenstein (1996) develops a model that includes visceral influences—such as hunger, thirst, pain, and stress—in an individual's instantaneous utility function. An advantage of this model over the present-biased model described above (also referred to as hyperbolic or quasi-hyperbolic discounting models) is that it allows a broader range of situ-ations to trigger present-biased behavior. At sufficient levels, visceral factors can create discrepancies between intended and actual behavior because an individual becomes unwilling to give up a good that alleviates the effects of a visceral influence in exchange for other goods that do not. For example, a man dying of thirst is unlikely to trade a glass of water for anything. This causes a collapsing of one's time perspective toward the present. Also, the discrepancy between the actual and desired value placed on a particular good or activity is assumed to increase with the intensity of the immediate good-relevant visceral factors.

To represent the influence of visceral factors on behavior, Loewenstein develops a representation of preferences that includes a set of variables, α_{ti}, which represent how changing levels of the visceral factors affect intertemporal utility:

$$U=\Sigma_t u(x_{t1},\ldots,x_{tn}, \alpha_{t1},\ldots\alpha_{tn}, t),$$

where U represents total utility experienced at time t, ($x_{t1},\ldots,x_{tn}$) is a vector of consumption goods, and ($\alpha_{t1},\ldots\alpha_{tn}$) is a vector of visceral factors, such as hours of food deprivation, experienced at time t. This model assumes prefer-ences are separable temporally so that visceral factors experienced at time t only influence the value of goods consumed at that same time. It is also assumed that visceral factors can be partitioned into subsets that infl uence only a single consumption variable. In the simplest case, each consumption variable x_i is influenced by at most one α_I, and can be represented as follows:

$$U=\Sigma_t u(v_1 (x_{t1}, \alpha_{t1}, t),\ldots v_n (x_{tn}, \alpha_{tn}, t)),$$

where $v_1()$ is the value of consuming x_{t1} at time t in the presence of some visceral factor α_{t1}. Each v_i function is assumed to be increasing in the good offered, decreasing in time delay, and either increasing or decreasing in α_{ti}. Also, x_{ti} and α_{ti} are assumed to be complements. For example, hunger can be argued to improve the enjoyment of eating food, but can make you feel worse when there is none available. In short, this model explicitly assumes that consumer choices will be significantly affected by strong visceral factors.

This model can illuminate how and why certain situations give rise to seemingly inconsistent food choices. Under a more neutral state, an individual may choose to consume the types and quantities of foods that are consistent with his or her long-term health objectives. As visceral factors intensify, however, the value of current utility increases relative to the value of future utility and the consumption of goods that provide immediate gratifi cation will be consumed in greater amounts than when visceral factors are less intense.

Theoretical Model

For this study, we use a relatively simple, two-period utility maximization problem that incorporates Loewenstein's visceral factors approach. Although a dynamic model may be more realistic, the general insights derived from a two-period model are the same. We assume that consumers make consump-tion decisions on a per meal basis and discount future well-being by some factor, δ, that is strictly less than one. In both the current and future periods, utility is derived from food (*F*), a composite nonfood item (N), and the individual's health status (*H*). For simplicity, we assume strong separability between food and nonfood, such that the utility received from food is not influenced by the amount of nonfood at that time. An individual's level of health, however, is assumed to complement both food and nonfood consump-tion. We also assume the utility function to be continuous, twice continu-ously differentiable, strictly increasing, and strictly concave in health, food, and nonfood items.

A vector of relevant visceral factors (α) experienced at the time an individual makes his or her consumption decision influences the level of utility received at that time. To isolate the effects of visceral factors on food consumption decisions, it is assumed that α influences only the utility derived from food consumed at that time. Holding all else constant, we assume that increasing visceral factors, such as the level of hunger experienced at the current time, will increase the marginal utility from food consumption so that an individual will require more food to provide the same level of utility compared to some neutral level of hunger. Thus, food and hunger are assumed to be comple-ments. Individuals are assumed to be naive and treat these visceral factors as exogenous[3] so that utility in both periods is derived from consumption of nonfood items, food (which is influenced by visceral impacts), and one's current level of health.

$$U = U_1(F(F_1; \alpha_1), N_1, H_1 + \delta U_2 (F(F_2; \alpha_2), N_2, H_2). \quad (1)$$

To isolate how individuals choose to balance immediate gratifi cation from food against possible future health implications of these decisions, we assume that one's current health is a function of his or her past dietary choices. For simplicity, we also assume that only less healthful foods have a positive impact on current utility from food and that these same foods have a negative impact on future health. How much an individual knows about health and nutrition (η) is assumed to affect how well he or she translates poor dietary choices into future health effects. Individuals who know more about the links between diet, nutrition, and health perceive a greater health impact from an unhealthy diet than individuals who know little about diet and health. This then leads to the following health production function:

$$H_t = H_t\,(F_{t\text{-}1};\, \eta_{t\text{-}1}) \qquad t = 1{,}2. \tag{2}$$

Finally, in both the current and future periods, an individual faces the following budget constraint:

$$P_{Nt}\,N_t + P_{Ft}\,F_t = \mathrm{Y}_t \qquad t = 1{,}2, \tag{3}$$

where P_{Nt} is the price of nonfood items, P_{Ft} is the price of food, and Y_t is the individual's income. Substituting the health production function (2) into (1), the Lagrangian for this two-period optimization problem can be written as:

$$\begin{aligned} L = {} & U_1(F(F_1;a_1), N_1, H_1\,(F_0; h_0)) + dU_2\,(F(F_2;\, a_2), N_2, H_2\,(F_1;h_1)) \\ & + l_1(Y_1 - P_{F1}\,F_1 - P_{N1}\,N_1) + l_2\,(Y_2 - P_{F2}\,F_2 - P_{N2}\,N_2). \end{aligned} \tag{4}$$

The first-order conditions for optimal consumption of unhealthful foods and nonfood items (F_1, N_1) at time 1 are:

$$L_{F1} = U_{1F1} + dU_{2H2}\,H_{2F1} - l_1\,P_{F1} = 0 \tag{5a}$$

$$L_{N1} = U_{1N1} - l_1\,P_{N1} = 0 \tag{5b}$$

$$L_{l1} = Y_1 - P_{F1}\,F_1 - P_{N1}\,N_1 = 0, \tag{5c}$$

where U_{1F1} and U_{1N1} are the current marginal utilities from food and nonfood consumed in the fi rst period, U_{2H2} is the marginal utility from health experienced in period 2, H_{2F1} is the marginal impact of the current period's poor food choices on next period's health, and $l_1$is the current marginal utility of wealth. For simplicity, we normalize prices and set P_{N1} equal to one. To be certain that these values of F_1, N_1 yield optimal values, we require the following condition to hold:

$$|dU_{2H2H2}\, H_{2F1}| < |\, (P_F)^2 U_{1N1N1} + U_{1F1F1} + dU_{2H2} H_{2F1F1}|. \tag{6}$$

Condition (6), along with Cramer's rule, can be used to determine how F_1 will change with specific parameters, such as current visceral infl uences and dietary awareness, and how the effect of dietary awareness on unhealthful food choices will change with the intensity of visceral infl uences.[4]

Proposition 1:

$$\partial F_1 / \partial \alpha_1 > 0$$

Increasing visceral factors in the current period will cause an individual to choose more unhealthful foods at that time.

Differentiating equations 5a-c with respect to a_1, rewriting the system of equations in matrix form, and solving this system of three equations using Cramer's rule, we find that the optimal choice of unhealthful foods will increase in the presence of relevant visceral factors as long as food and visceral factors (hunger, stress) are complements. Since $U_{1F1a1} > 0$ is true by construction, proposition 1 holds.

Proposition 2:

$$\partial F_1 / \partial \eta_1 < 0$$

Increasing an individual's awareness about the negative impact of poor dietary choices on future health will cause him or her to eat fewer unhealthful foods.

Using the same technique and differentiating the fi rst-order conditions with respect to h_1 and again solving this system of equations via Cramer's rule, individuals with higher levels of health information will choose fewer unhealthful foods as long as $U_{2H2}H_{2F1h1} < 0$. We assume that an individual who is more informed about the links between diet and health will be better able to assess the negative health effects of his or her poor food choices, thus $H_{2F1\eta1} < 0$.[5] This then ensures that an individual will respond to an increase in health information by choosing fewer unhealthful foods for current consumption.

Proposition 3:

$$\partial^2 F_1 / \partial\eta_1\partial\alpha_1 = \partial^2 F_1 / \partial\alpha_1\partial\eta_1 < 0$$

As visceral factors increase at a given time or eating occasion, an individual's health information will have less impact on his or her food choice. Alternatively, individuals with higher levels of health and dietary information will be less affected by visceral factors than individuals with lower levels of dietary information.

Again, differentiating the first-order conditions with respect to η_1 and then differentiating each with respect to α_1, we fi nd that $\partial^2 F_1 / \partial\eta_1\partial\alpha_1$ is less than zero as long as

$$\left|\delta U_{2H2} H_{2F1F1\eta1} \partial F_1 / \partial\alpha_1\right| < \left|U_{1F1F\alpha1} \partial F_1 / \partial\eta_1 + \delta U_{2H2H2} H_{2F1\eta1} \partial F_1 / \partial\alpha_1\right|. \quad (7)$$

Our goal is to sign comparative statics for a typical individual, not all mathematically possible utility and health production functions. We therefore make additional, but reasonable, assumptions. The first is that the health production function is convex—the negative effect of poor food choices on health increases as an individual's health status decreases. Another is that better dietary information is assumed to simply shift the health production function inward while leaving the rate at which poor food choices affect overall health unchanged. Thus, $H_{2F1F1\eta1} = 0$. Similarly, we can assume that increasing visceral factors simply causes an outward shift in the utility one receives from food. We can also assume that increasing visceral factors causes the marginal utility received from food to increase, but at a decreasing rate. Simply put, as visceral factors like hunger or stress intensify, additional amounts of food increase overall utility at lower rates. This conforms with the idea that many people tend to make poorer food choices when hungry or under stress. As long as we assume that $U_{1F1F\alpha1} \leq 0$, condition (7) will hold. This in turn implies that $\partial^2 F_1 / \partial\eta_1\partial\alpha_1 < 0$.

Empirical Implications and Economic Model

The theoretical model implies that demand for unhealthful foods at time t will be a function of income, prices, visceral factors, and health at time t. To test whether visceral influences weaken the impact of health information on food choices, we also include the interaction of visceral factors and nutrition information. Empirically, demand for unhealthful food in the current period can be specified as follows:

$$F_{it} = \beta' X_{it} + u_i + e_{it}, \tag{8}$$

where F_{it} is the amount of unhealthful food individual i consumes at each eating occasion t, X_{it} is a vector of the aforementioned parameters—income, prices, current health status, visceral factors—and the interaction of dietary information and visceral infl uences, u_i is the individual effect, and e_{it} is the individual, time-specific error term. If there is more than one observation for an individual, as there is in this study, ordinary least squares (OLS) estimates will yield inefficient parameter estimates if the error terms are correlated across observations for a given individual.

A random-effects (RE) model will yield efficient and consistent estimates as long as the individual specific disturbance (u_i) is uncorrelated with the other regressors, X_{it}. However, given the interdependence of current health, dietary awareness, and food choices, this condition will likely not be met. For example, an individual recently diagnosed with diabetes may be more aware of diet and nutrition. This same person would also have greater incentives to improve his or her diet quality and manage the timing of his or her meals. Not accounting for this health condition in the RE estimator would then bias estimates on both the impact of dietary awareness and the interval between meals.

As such, a fixed-effects (FE) model, as specified below, will yield consistent estimates as long as the remaining individual-specifi c, time-specifi c distur-bance (e_{it}) is also uncorrelated with the regressors (Green, 1990):

$$(F_{it} - \overline{F}_i) = \beta' (X_{it} - \overline{X}_i) + (e_{it} - \overline{e}_{it}), \tag{9}$$

where F_i, X_i, and e_i represent individual averages. Continuing with the previous example, a fixed-effects estimator allows one to tease out the impact of time-varying variables, such as the interval between meals. In this case, the FE estimates would measure the impact of meal timing on diet quality for a given individual with specific health conditions and dietary aware-ness. If, however, the time-specific disturbances are also correlated with the regressors, a fixed-effects model with instrumental variables (FE-IV) can be used to obtain unbiased estimates (Evans et al., 1993). Theoretically, there is reason to suspect that the error terms will be correlated with the explanatory variables because some visceral factors, such as how long one goes between meals, are arguably endogenous and/or possibly measured with error. Thus, we attempt to circumvent this issue through the use of instrumental variables.

We use Stata 9.0 for our empirical analysis. Specifically, we use xtset to identify the nature of our panel data. We specify each individual as the panel variable and each meal as the time variable. We then use xtivreg, a fixed-effects instrumental variable (FE-IV) estimator that uses a two-stage, least-squares within estimator. We also employed random-effects (RE) and fixed-effects (FE) estimators, using generalized least squares. However, the Hausman test statistics indicate that these results were biased.[6] We therefore only describe variables used in the FE-IV estimation and limit our discussion and presentation of these FE-IV results.

DATA

The data for this study come from the USDA's 1994-96 Continuing Survey of Food Intakes by Individuals (CSFII) and the companion Diet and Health Knowledge Survey (DHKS). Through dietary recalls, the CSFII contains information on the foods and nutrients consumed over 2 nonconsecutive days. The DHKS provides information on peoples' attitudes and knowledge about diet, health, and nutrition. In each CSFII household, the DHKS was administered to only one adult over 20 years old who reported at least 1 day of food intake. To maintain a clear link among food consumption, visceral influences, and dietary awareness, this analysis includes only individuals who were also given the DHKS. In total, we have information on 5,645 indi-viduals who reported an average of 6.4 eating occasions, for a total sample of 36,312 observations. Descriptions of variables used in the empirical analysis and their summary statistics are in table 1.

Dependent Variables

Calories

For the empirical analysis, the first step is to provide a suitable and measurable definition of unhealthful food choices made at each eating occasion. As energy imbalance and large portion sizes are often linked to weight gain and ultimately poor health, one measure used in this study is the number of calories consumed at an eating occasion. As such, one dependent variable is the share of recommended calories consumed at a specifi c eating occasion.[7] It is the number of calories an individual consumes divided by an individual's daily estimated energy requirement (EER), multiplied by 100. An individual's EER is calculated using the equations from the Institute of Medicine (2002), which is a function of an individual's age, gender, height, weight, and physical activity.[8] As an example, if an individual's daily EER is 2,000 calories and he or she consumes 500 calories at breakfast, then the dependent variable at that eating occasion is 25.

Healthy Meal Index

Low nutrient intake is also correlated with poor health and weight outcomes. Ideally, we would like a measure of nutrient intake per unit of energy consumed, such as nutrient density relative to energy density. At this time, however, there is no standard definition for this measure. To deal with this issue, we try three separate measures of nutrient quality. The first makes use of calculations from an individual's Healthy Eating Index for 1994-96. We refer to this measure as the HEI score. This index, which ranges from 0 to 100, summarizes how well an individual's daily food intake conforms to the 1995 *Dietary Guidelines for Americans*. The components of this index are an individual's intake of fruits, vegetables, grains, dairy prod-ucts, meat, fat, saturated fat, sodium, and cholesterol (Bowman et al., 1998). To make this measure usable on a per-meal basis, we use a SAS program (available upon request from the USDA) to calculate an individual's daily HEI score.[9] We then augment the program to calculate what each person's daily score would have been in the absence of each eating occasion on a specifi c day.

The dependent variable at each eating occasion is the difference between what that individual's HEI score actually was on that day of intake and what it would have been in the absence of that specific eating occasion. For example, if an individual's HEI score on the first day of intake was 65 and that score would have been 60 had he or she not eaten breakfast that day, the dependent variable for that individual at that breakfast eating occasion would have a value of 5. Thus, higher values for this variable represent meal choices that are more nutritious. We refer to this variable as the Healthy Meal Index (HMI) to be clear that it is meant to gauge the nutritional quality of each eating occasion, whereas the HEI measures diet quality over an entire day.

Table 1. Variables, Definitions and Summary Statistics

Variable	Definition	Mean (standard deviation)
Calories	Percent of daily energy requirements consumed at eating occasion	22.26 (19.68)
Healthy Meal Index (HMI)	How much higher HEI score (0-100 points) would have been without eating occasion	3.44 (6.21)
HMI2005	HEI 2005 density score at eating occasion (0-100 points)	37.70 (13.22)
SOFAAS per meal	Calories from solid fats, alcohol, and added sugar (0-20 points)	10.29 (9.30)
Interval	Hours elapsed between current and previous eating occasion	3.66 (2.22)
Share restaurant food	Share of food from restaurant (calories)	13.39 (33.51)
Brunch	1 if classified as brunch; 0 otherwise	0.01
Lunch	1 if classified as lunch; 0 otherwise	0.22
Dinner	1 if classified as dinner; 0 otherwise	0.30
Snack	1 if classified as snack; 0 otherwise	0.42
Weekend	1 if dietary recall occurred on a weekend; 0 otherwise	0.26
Knowledge	Score on dietary knowledge assessment (0-100)	71.71 (13.35)
Work hours	Number of hours worked in previous week	23.46 (23.39)
Interaction: Interval* knowledge	Interval*score on dietary knowledge assessment (0-100)	260.51 (164.64)
Interaction: Interval*work hours	Interval*Number of hours worked in previous week	86.40 (117.23)
Interaction: Share-fafh*knowledge	Share of restaurant food*score on dietary knowledge assessment	954.42 (2,434.42)
Interaction: Sharefafh*work hours	Share of restaurant food*Number of hours worked in previous week	400.55 (1,314.51)

Each variable's standard deviation is listed below its mean for all continuous variables. Sample size is 36,312, with 5,645 individuals who report an average of 6.43 eating occasions.

Each of the 10 HEI components falls within the range of 1 to 10. Thus, someone who ate more than his or her recommended levels of fruit or vegetables could not score bonus points by doing so. Similarly, there are limits to "penalties" for overconsumption of salt, cholesterol, fat, and saturated fat. This top and bottom coding within components enables the HEI score to be more than a simple linear function of each meal's score. In the absence of such coding, however, the sum of HMI scores over an entire day would equal an individual's daily HEI score.

Healthy Meal Index, 2005

In 2005, the USDA and Department of Health and Human Services updated the *Dietary Guidelines for Americans*. More recently, the USDA has created the HEI-2005 (Guenther et al., 2007), which refl ects the 2005 *Dietary Guidelines* and addresses some shortcomings of the HEI score. For example, it did not assess caloric intake or excesses of some components such as added sugars or alcohol. Also, the HEI score did not differentiate between types of vegetables, grains, or fats. As such, a serving of french fries and a serving of kale contributed equally to an individual's HEI score.

Intuitively, it seems better to gauge the links between dietary knowledge in 1994-96 and dietary intake in 1994-96 using the HEI score derived from the dietary guidelines promoted during this same time. However, we also run estimates using a Healthy Meal Index based on the HEI-2005 score to see how visceral influences, dietary knowledge, and meal location infl uence alternative measures of diet quality. The 12 components that make up the HEI-2005 score are total fruit, whole fruit, total vegetables, dark green and orange vegetables and legumes, total grains, whole grains, milk, meat and beans, oils, saturated fat, sodium, and calories from solid fats, alcohol, and added sugar (SoFAAS). Scoring for 10 of the 12 components is based on caloric density—either cups, grams, or ounce equivalents per 1,000 grams. Scoring for sodium and SoFAAS is calculated as a percent of energy. As such, it is easier to translate this daily measure into a per meal measure. We simply calculate each of the 12 components using the calories consumed at that meal instead of the total calories consumed over the entire day. We refer to this measure as the Healthy Meal Index 2005 (HMI-2005).

Calories from Solid Fats, Alcohol, and Added Sugar (SoFAAS)

The twelfth component—SoFAAS—measures discretionary calories. Excess calories and energy imbalance are the cause of weight gain, and limiting discretionary calories is an effective way to reduce caloric intake without necessarily reducing nutrient intake. We run a final model that estimates how visceral influences and other explanatory variables influence intake of discre-tionary calories, or SoFAAS, at a meal.

Explanatory Variables

According to the theoretical model, per-meal food demand will be a function of food prices, income, current health, and meal-specific visceral factors such as hunger.[10] Although the CSFII does not explicitly ask individuals how hungry they were at each eating occasion, it does provide information on the time elapsed between eating occasions. We therefore use the interval between meals, measured in hours, as a proxy for an individual's level of hunger at a specific eating occasion. This effect may change after longer periods without food, so we also include a quadratic term for the interval between meals.

We include the type of eating occasion (breakfast, lunch, dinner, or snack) and whether or not the dietary recall occurred on a weekend or weekday, as these variables may also affect individuals' food choices. The data on dietary intake come from 2 nonconsecutive days, so there are two observations each day (the first eating occasion) where it is not possible to calculate the interval between meals. Rather than lose these observations, we assign the mean interval between meals for each individual and use that as the level of hunger for the first eating occasion (Cohen et al., 2003).

To test the proposition that dietary awareness will have less infl uence on food choice in the presence of strong visceral influences, we include an interactive term to estimate the effects of dietary knowledge as hunger increases. Responses from the DHKS are used to create an index to measure knowledge about health and nutrition for each individual. One-third of this knowledge index is created by summing the number of questions an individual answered correctly about the links between diet and health.[11] Specifi cally, individuals were asked if they knew how many servings of fruit, vegetables, meat, dairy, and grains they should consume each day. They scored one point for each correct answer. Another third of this index is created from scoring correct answers about the amounts of cholesterol, fat, and saturated fat in specifi c foods. The remaining third of the information index comes from the DHKS questions on the importance of certain dietary practices, such as eating enough fruits, vegetables, and fiber; limiting intake of fat, cholesterol, saturated fat, salt, and sugar; and maintaining a healthy body weight.

Where an individual makes his or her food choices may affect the types and amounts of foods consumed. To gauge this effect, we calculate the share of calories consumed at each meal that come from a restaurant (restaurants with table service, fast-food places, pizza places, and bars/taverns).[12] We also estimate if the effect of dietary knowledge wanes when consuming foods away from home because typically there is less health information about foods purchased at restaurants.

Finally, stress of time pressures associated with work and family requirements may be a visceral influence that, like hunger, affects food choice. As a proxy for work requirements, we use the number of hours worked in the previous week. Although this specific variable is not in our empirical estimation, we do include an interactive term to determine whether hunger has a stronger effect on individuals who are more time constrained through work. We also interact *hours worked* with food away from home to estimate if time stresses increase an individual's vulnerability to certain pitfalls of eating away from home, such as an expanded array of unhealthy food choices or less information about diet/nutrition.

Instrumental Variables

Using a fixed-effects estimator should drastically reduce the correla-tion between the disturbance terms and the other explanatory variables. However, it is possible that the variable we use to proxy an individual's level of hunger may be correlated with some unobserved time-varying factor. Obtaining unbiased, efficient estimates requires that the additional variables be both relevant and independent. Because we assume a fi xed-effects estimator, the instruments also need to vary across observations for a single individual. Therefore, some time-invariant variables, such as health conditions of other family members, are not viable options. In the fixed-effects model, there are four variables that are created using the interval between meals (hunger, hunger squared, the interaction of hunger with dietary knowledge, and the interaction of hunger with hours worked).[13] Thus, these variables may be correlated with the individual-specifi c, time-varying error term. One possible instrument is to use the time of day an eating occasion occurred. The time of day is exogenous—while people may choose how long they go between meals, they do not choose the actual time of day. However, certain times, such as 4 p.m., may be more correlated with longer intervals between meals compared to 12:30 p.m. Following the technique developed by Arellano and Bond (1991), we also use lags of the endogenous variables as instruments.[14] How long one has gone between meals previously is likely to be correlated with how long one has gone between meals at present. However, feeling hungry at lunch should not influence how hungry one feels at dinner.[15]

In summary, we employ a fixed-effects estimator with instrumental variables (FE-IV) described as follows:

$$(F_{it} - \overline{F}_i) = \beta'(X_{it} - \overline{X}_i) + \gamma'(\alpha_{it} - \overline{\alpha}_i) + (e_{it} - \overline{e}_i) \tag{10a}$$

$$(\alpha_{it} - \overline{\alpha}_i) = \xi' + (Z_{it} - \overline{Z}_i) + (\varepsilon_{it} - \overline{\varepsilon}_i). \tag{10b}$$

We use four different dependent variables: the share of an individual's recommended daily caloric intake consumed at an eating occasion; the difference between what an individual's HEI score would have been in the absence of that specific eating occasion and what it was on that day of intake (HMI); the HEI-2005 density score per eating occasion (HMI-2005); and the share of discretionary calories consumed at each eating occasion (SoFAAS). In each model, we include proxies for visceral factors—stress and hunger—and the interaction of these visceral factors with nutrition information as explanatory variables.

RESULTS

Estimation results, the Hausman test statistic comparing the FE-IV results to the FE results, and the Godfrey-Hutton test for overidentifi cation are reported in table 2. In three out of the four models, the high values on the Hausman tests indicate that there are systematic differences between the instrumental (IV) and non-IV estimates. For estimation of the HMI-2005 scores, we cannot reject the hypothesis that the FE-IV estimates do not differ significantly from the FE estimates. However, the results of the FE-IV model are still consistent under the null hypothesis. Thus, we focus on the FE-IV estimates and discuss only those results that are statistically significant at the 5-percent level or above. However, we are more confident of our model's estimating changes in calories and changes in diet quality using the HMI score because the higher values of the Godfrey-Hutton test indicate that the models for SoFAAS and HMI-2005 may be overidentified, meaning that not all of the instruments are valid.

The interaction terms make it difficult to judge the impact of time between meals and eating food away from home by simply looking at the estimated coefficients. Thus, we ran simulations using the sample means and changing variables of interest to measure the impact of changing specifi c variables.[16]

Table 2. Estimation Results

FE-IV Estimates[a]	Calories	Healthy Meal Index	Healthy Meal Index 2005	SOFAAS per meal
Parameter estimates (Standard errors)				
Interval	3.384** (1.637)	-1.417** (0.599)	-2.351* (1.227)	-3.463*** (0.945)
$Interval^2$	-0.305*** (0.0957)	0.109*** (0.0353)	0.137* (0.0718)	0.313*** (0.0553)
Share restaurant food	0.133*** (0.0185)	0.0216*** (0.00686)	0.0249* (0.0140)	-0.0296*** (0.0108)
Brunch	2.935** (1.208)	0.668 (0.444)	-0.310 (0.906)	-0.0938 (0.698)
Lunch	5.494*** (0.931)	2.866*** (0.342)	2.869*** (0.703)	0.330 (0.542)
Dinner	12.46*** (0.947)	4.843*** (0.348)	4.658*** (0.713)	-0.412 (0.549)
Snack	-8.103*** (0.564)	-0.0609 (0.207)	-4.961*** (0.426)	-0.957*** (0.328)
Interval*knowledge	0.00784 (0.0176)	0.00453 (0.00639)	0.00715 (0.0131)	-0.00613 (0.0101)
Interval*work hours	0.0289*** (0.0102)	-0.00782** (0.00376)	-0.00402 (0.00767)	-0.0141** (0.00591)
Sharefafh*knowledge	-0.000730*** (0.000247)	-0.000340*** (0.0000914)	-0.000670*** (0.000187)	-0.0000397 (0.000144)
Sharefafh*work hours	-0.000610*** (0.000139)	0.00000157 (0.0000515)	0.000286*** (0.000105)	0.000268*** (0.0000811)
Weekend	1.431*** (0.246)	0.00916 (0.0904)	-0.795*** (0.185)	-0.628*** (0.142)
Constant	8.153*** (1.846)	4.085*** (0.678)	42.85*** (1.384)	21.05*** (1.066)
Overall R^2	.2911	0.0724	0.0704	0.0159
Sample size	35,151	35,835	35,452	35,452
Hausman Test Statistic[b]	32.32***	25.95***	14.60	66.36***
Godfrey-Hutton J-statistic[c]	7.03	0.00	10.64**	31.91***

Note: Instruments: Time of eating occasion, lagged values of each endogenous variable. *** p<0.01, ** p<0.05, * p<0.1

[a] Endogenous variables: Interval, Interval2, Interval*knowledge, and Interval*work hours.

[b] H0: Difference between FE and FE-IV estimates is not systematic.

[c] H0: All of the instruments are valid.

Our results indicate that increasing the interval between meals will have a significant impact on consumption volume and diet quality. In general, as the time interval between eating occasions increases, the calories consumed at the latter meal increase, nutritional quality (HMI, HMI-2005) of that meal decreases, and consumption of discretionary calories (SoFAAS) rises. Our estimates suggest that going 5 hours between meals instead of 4 adds about 52 calories for someone on a diet of 2,000 calories per day; extending that interval from 4 to 6 hours would add about 91 calories. The impact on diet quality is also significant. Recall that a higher HMI or HMI-2005 implies a more nutritious meal or snack and a higher SoFAAS score indicates fewer discretionary calories consumed. Using the HMI score, going from 4 to 5 hours is estimated to reduce diet quality by 0.4 point, while going from 4 to 6 hours lowers this score by 0.6 point. Using the HMI-2005 score, these same changes in the timing between meals lead to a 0.75- and 1.25-point reduc-tion in HMI-2005 score and a 1.7- and 2.7-point reduction in the per-meal SoFAAS score (out of a total score of 20).

The location at which someone makes his or her food choices (share restau-rant food) and when these choices are made significantly affect what and how much is consumed. Not surprisingly, people are estimated to eat more caloric meals when eating foods from a restaurant compared with foods prepared at home—about 107 more calories per meal. They also consume more discre-tionary calories (solid fats, alcohol, and added sugars) when eating meals away from home—our estimates indicate an individual's SoFAAS score would fall by 2 points when eating away from home.

A surprising finding, however, is that overall diet quality is estimated to significantly improve when eating foods prepared away from home. The HMI estimates suggest that meals away from home would add about 5 points to one's total daily HEI score, whereas the HMI-2005 suggests a meal away from home would add 3 points compared with meals at home.

People eat more at brunch, lunch, and dinner than at breakfast. Lunch and dinner are also estimated to significantly add to daily diet quality—both the HMI and HMI-2005 scores indicate lunches were almost 3 points higher than breakfast, and dinners were over 4 points higher than breakfast. Food consumed as snacks is significantly smaller compared to other eating occa-sions, but may lower diet quality—both the HMI-2005 and the SoFAAS were significantly lower for snacks.

Examining the interaction of dietary information and visceral factors provides mixed support for our theoretical hypotheses. In all cases, the coef-ficient on the interval*knowledge variable is not significant. One way to interpret this would be that dietary knowledge has no impact on one's reac-tion to longer intervals between meals. Or, the length of the interval between meals may have no effect on the relationship between dietary knowledge and food choices.

In support of our hypothesis, however, we find that our proxy for time pres-sures interacts significantly with the interval between meals (interval*work hours). Our estimates suggest that people who work more hours in a week are also more influenced by the interval between meals than those who work fewer hours. As an individual who works more hours in a week goes longer between meals, he or she will choose a meal that is signifi cantly higher in calories, higher in discretionary calories, and lower in diet quality, as measured by the HMI-2005. At 4 hours between meals, an individual who works 40 hours a week is estimated to eat about 20 percent more calories than someone who is not employed. At 8 hours between meals, the fully employed individual is estimated to eat nearly 40 percent more calories than someone who is not employed.

We also find that a situational change in caloric intake and diet quality is more pronounced among individuals who are less informed about diet and nutrition. A person with a knowledge score of 50 is estimated to increase per-meal caloric intake by about 28 percent when eating away from home, while a person whose score is 100 points is estimated to eat about only 12 percent more calories when eating away from home. Using the 1994-96 measure of diet quality, we find that increasing health information is associated with making healthier choices, both at home and away from home. When eating at home, a person with a knowledge score of 100 scores about 1 point higher on the HMI than someone with a score of 50. However, this difference falls to 0.8 point when eating away from home. This may be because informa-tion about nutrient content is more difficult to obtain on foods prepared away from home.

However, when using the HMI-2005 to measure diet quality, we fi nd that diet quality responds differently to knowledge depending on whether a person is eating at home or away from home. At home, a person who scored 100 on the knowledge index scored about 1.43 points higher than someone who scored 50 on the knowledge index. Away from home, however, the person with a perfect knowledge score was estimated to score nearly 2 points lower on the HMI-2005 than someone who scored 50 on the knowledge index. However, it should be noted that in all cases—calories, HMI, and HMI-2005—the estimated effect of this variable is relatively small and not statistically significant.

Contrary to our theoretical hypothesis, the interaction between hours worked and eating away from home was estimated to significantly improve diet choices (share restaurant food*work hours). While individuals who are fully employed are again estimated to eat more calories at each meal than individ-uals who are not, this difference shrinks as the share of food away from home increases. When eating at home, individuals who work 40 hours a week are estimated to eat about 92 calories more per meal than those who worked 0 hours. When eating away from home, this difference shrinks to 43 calories per meal. Thus, we find that people who report working more hours away from home are also better able to make healthful choices when eating out, perhaps because it is something they do more regularly.

CONCLUSION

The sharp increase in overweight and obesity among Americans has occurred concurrently with increased awareness and publicity regarding the benefi ts of a healthy lifestyle. Examining this phenomenon provides an opportunity to incorporate elements of behavioral economics into consumer food choice analysis. In such analysis, both long-term health objectives and short-term situational factors drive individuals' food choices.

The interaction among these long-term goals and short-term situations can then explain seemingly time-inconsistent choices. The resulting theoretical model predicts that when individuals are experiencing strong visceral infl u-ences, such as hunger or stress, their information about health and nutri-tion will have less impact on their actual food choices. It also predicts that individuals who are less informed about health and nutrition, or consume more food prepared away from home, will be more likely to eschew their longrun goals when faced with short-term situational factors such as hunger. The value of this model is that it explicitly identifies elements that increase demand for goods and services that offer more immediate gratifi cation.

The empirical results confirm that incorporating findings from behavioral economics into the analysis of nutrient intake illuminates how situational factors and long-term health objectives affect our food choices. Specifi cally, when individuals extend the period between meals or consume more of their food away from home, they are significantly more likely to consume more calories at each eating occasion. Going longer intervals between meals, especially when working more hours in a week, also reduces the diet quality of specifi c meals.

This study also suggests that in the face of visceral influences, one's intentions may have little to no impact on actual food choices. As people change their dietary goals based on prevailing nutritional beliefs, situational factors like hunger and time pressures will continue to interfere with their long-term health objectives. Making specific reference to such situations and suggesting ways to mitigate their effects should enhance the usefulness of educational campaigns designed to improve diet quality. For example, encouraging consumers to take more active control in limiting the interval between meals and choosing nutrient-dense snacks, such as fruits and vegetables, may help them better align their intentions to eat well with their actual behavior. Limiting intake of foods prepared away from home is also estimated to significantly decrease caloric consumption. Thus, another possibility would be to encourage individuals to plan ahead or seek out information about nutrient and caloric content of foods prepared away from home.

REFERENCES

Abdulai, A. & Aubert, D. (2004). "A Cross-Section Analysis of Household Demand for Food and Nutrients in Tanzania," *Agricultural Economics, 31,* 67-79.

Ainslie, G. & Haslam, N. (1992). "Hyperbolic Discounting" and "Self-Control," in *Choice Over Time*, George Loewenstein and John Elster (eds.). New York: Russel Sage Foundation.

Akerlof, G. A. (1991). "Procrastination and Obedience," *American Economic Review, 81(2)*, 1-19.

Ackman, D. (2005). "Big News on Fat Front," *Forbes Magazine*. January 12.

Arrelano, M. & Bond, S. (1991). "Some Tests of Specification for Panel Data: Monte Carlo Evidence and an Application to Employment Equations," *The Review of Economic Studies, 58(2)*, 277-297.

Barrett, C. B. (2002). "Food Security and Food Assistance Programs," in *Handbook of Agricultural Economics, Volume 2*, B. Gardner and G. Rausser (eds.). Elsevier Sciences.

Behrman, J. R. & Deolalikar, A. B. (1990). "The Intrahousehold Demand for Nutrients in Rural South India: Individual Estimates, Fixed Effects and Permanent Income," *The Journal of Human Resources, 25(4),* 665-696.

Bellisle, F. & Rolland-Cachera, M. F. (2001). "How Sugar-Containing Drinks Might Increase Adiposity in Children," *The Lancet, 357*, 490-491.

Bhargava, A., Franzini, L. & Narendranathan, W. (1982). "Serial Correlation and the Fixed Effects Model," *The Review of Economic Studies, 49(4)*, 533-549.

Bowman, S. A., Lino, M., Gerrior, S. A. & Bastiosis, P. (1998). *The Healthy Eating Index:1994-1996.* U.S. Department of Agriculture, Center for Nutrition Policy and Promotion. CNPP-5. http://www.cnpp.usda.gov/hei94-96.PDF

Cawley, J. (2004). "An Economic Framework for Understanding Physical Activity and Eating Behaviors," *American Journal of Preventive Medicine, 27(3S)*, 117-125.

Centers for Disease Control and Prevention. 2003."1991–2001 Prevalence of Obesity Among U.S. Adults, by Characteristics." http://www.cdc.gov/nccdphp/dnpa/obesity/trend/prev_char.htm

________. 2005. "Chronic Disease Overview." http://www.cdc.gov/nccdphp/overview.htm

Cohen, J., Cohen, P., West, S. & Aiken, L. (2003). *Applied Multiple Regression/Correlation Analysis for the Behavioral Sciences* (3rd ed.). Mahwah, NJ: Erlbaum.

Cutler, D. M., Glaeser, E. L. & Shapiro, J. M. (2003). "Why Have Americans Become More Obese?" NBER Working Paper 9446. http://www.nber.org/papers/w9446

Evans, W. N., Froeb, L. M. & Werden, G. J. (1993). "Endogeneity in the Concentration-Price Relationship: Causes, Consequences and Cures," *The Journal of Industrial Economics, 41(4)*, 431-438.

Food Institute Reports. 2004-2005. *Weekly Newsletter of The Food Institute*, Elmwood Park, NJ, March 10, 2004, and January 31, 2005, editions.

Food Marketing Institute. 2001a "Reaching Out to the Whole Health Consumer," *Prevention Magazine*. Rodale Incorporated.

___________. 2002. *Shopping for Health*, Washington, DC. http://www.fmi.org

Frederick, S., Loewenstein, G. & O'Donoghue, T. (2002). "Time Discounting and Time Preference: A Critical Review," *Journal of Economic Literature, 40*, 351-401.

Green, W. H. (1990). *Econometric Analysis.* New York, Macmillan Publishing Company.

Grossman, M. (1972). "On the Concept of Health Capital and the Demand for Health," *The Journal of Political Economy, 80*, 223-225.

Guenther, P. M., Reedy, J., Krebs-Smith, S. M., Reeve, B. B. & Basiotis, P. P. (2007). *Development of the the Healthy Eating Index-2005: Technical*

Report. Center for Nutrition Policy and Promotion, U.S. Department of Agriculture.

Herman, C. P. & Polivy, J. (2003). "Dieting as an Exercise in Behavioral Economics," *Time and Decision.* George Lowenstein, Daniel Reed and Roy Baumeister (eds.), New York: Russel Sage Foundation.

Hoch, S. J. & Loewestein, G. F. (1991). "Time-Inconsistent Preferences and Consumer Self Control," *The Journal of Consumer Research, 17(4)*, 492-507.

Institute of Medicine of the National Academies. (2002). "Energy," *Dietary Reference Intakes for Energy, Carbohydrate, Fiber, Fat, Fatty Acids, Cholesterol, Protein, and Amino Acids (Macronutrients).* Washington, DC: The National Academies Press.

Kuchler, F. & Lin, B. H. (2002). "The Influence of Individual Choices and Attitudes on Adiposity," *International Journal of Obesity, 26*, 1017-1022.

Laibson, D. (2001). "A Cue-Theory of Consumption," *The Quarterly Journal of Economics, 116*, 81-119.

_______. 1997. "Golden Eggs and Hyperbolic Discounting," *Quarterly Journal of Economics, 112*, 443-477.

Lewbel, A. (1997). "Constructing Instruments for Regressions with Measurement Error when no Additional Data are Available, with an Application to Patents and R&D," *Econometrica, 65*, 1201-1213.

Loewenstein, G. (2000). "Emotions in Economic Theory and Economic Behavior," *The American Economic Review, 90(2)*, 426-432.

___________. (1996). "Out of Control: Visceral Influences on Behavior," *Organizational Behavior and Human Decision Processes, 65(3)*, 272-292.

Mancino, L. & Kinsey, J. (2004). *Diet Quality and Calories Consumed: The Impact of Being Hungrier, Busier, and Eating Out.* WP-04-02. The Food Industry Center, University of Minnesota.

Mullainathan, S. & Thaler, R. (2000). "Behavioral Economics." NBER Working Paper #7984.

O'Donoghue, T. & Rabin, M. (2001). "Choice and Procrastination," *Quarterly Journal of Economics, 116*, 121-160.

____________________. (1999). "Doing it Now or Later," *American Economic Review, 89*, 103-124.

Park, J. & Davis, G. C. (2001). "The Theory and Econometrics of Health Information in Cross-Sectional Nutrient Demand Analysis," *American Journal of Agricultural Economics, 83*, 840-851.

Pitt, M. M., Rosenzweig, M. R. & Hassan, N. (1990). "Productivity, Health and Inequality in the Intrahousehold Distribution of Food in Low-Income Countries," *The American Economic Review, 80(5)*, 1139-1156.

Read, D. & van Leeuwen, B. (1998). "Predicting Hunger: The Effects of Appetite and Delay on Choice," *Organizational Behavior and Human Decision Processes, 76(2)*, 189-205.

The Surgeon General's Call To Action To Prevent and Decrease Overweight and Obesity. 2001. *http://www.surgeongeneral.gov/news/* pressreleases/ pr_obesity.PDF .

Thaler, R. H. (1981). "Some Empirical Evidence on Dynamic Inconsistency," *Economic Letters, (8)*, 201-207.

Thaler R. H. & Shefrin, H. M. (1981)"An Economic Theory of Self Control," *Journal of Political Economy, 89(2)*, 392-410.

United States Department of Agriculture, Center for Nutrition Policy and Promotion (CNPP). 2006. "Development of MyPyramid," http://www.cnpp.usda.gov/MyPyramidDevelopment.htm.

United States Department of Agriculture. (2006). "USDA 2006 Budget Summary," http://www.usda.gov/agency/obpa/Budget-Summary/2006/FYbudsum.pdf

Variyam, J. N. (2003). *Factors Affecting the Macronutrient Intake of U.S. Adults*. U.S. Department of Agriculture, Economic Research Service, Technical Bulletin No. 1901.

Variyam, J. N., Blaylock, J. & Smallwood, D. (1995). *Modeling Nutrient Intake: The Role of Dietary Information*. U.S. Department of Agriculture, Economic Research Service, Technical Bulletin No. 1842.

_______(1996). "A Probit Latent Variable Model of Nutrition Information and Dietary Fiber Intake," *American Journal of Agricultural Economics, 78*, 628-639.

End Notes

[1] An individual is classified as obese if his or her body mass index (BMI), or ratio of one's weight in kilograms to one's squared height in meters, exceeds 30. An individual with a BMI between 25 and 30 is classified as overweight.

[2] See Frederick et al. (2003) for a full review.

[3] Treating visceral influences as en-dogenous would complicate the model without providing additional insights. Fully sophisticated individuals would control visceral influences such that their optimal choice of food would be the same as that under a state of neutral visceral influences. Loewenstein (1996, 2000) argues that while individuals do control their situations, they underesti-mate the effect that visceral infl uences will have in the future.

Thus, although our theoretical model could accom-modate this by allowing individuals to have an underestimated idea of their future visceral levels, the ultimate fi nd-ings of our model would be the same: As visceral factors increase, individu-als would consume more food and the strength of dietary information on guiding food choices would decline.

[4] A detailed account of the propositions and their proofs is available upon request.

[5] By assumption, information affects only how accurately one relates dietary choices to health outcomes. It does not have an impact on the level of enjoy-ment derived from health.

[6] We do not reject the null-hypothesis that the difference between the FE and FE-IV coefficients are not systematic for one model. However, even if the null hypothesis is rejected, FE-IV estimates are consistent.

[7] A potential weakness of looking at the relationship between meal timing and calories consumed on a per meal basis is that calories consumed at each meal may not adequately reflect total calories consumed over a day. Someone who frequently eats small meals could ultimately consume more total calories over the day. Using the same CSFII data and looking at calories consumed throughout the day, however, Mancino and Kinsey (2004) also found a positive and signifi cant cor-relation between time between meals and total calories consumed.

[8] In our calculations, we assume that all individuals are inactive because the activity data available in the CSFII are not precise enough to include as part of the EER calculation.

[9] The official HEI score also includes a variety component. However, it is very difficult to calculate the change in daily HEI score while including this component. For that reason, the HEI scores in this study only include 9 com-ponents. Thus, the range of scores is from 0 to 90. We feel this does not alter results dramatically, especially since the HEI-2005 score does not include a variety component.

[10] Because we do not discuss the results of the random effects (RE) estimates in the body of the paper, we do not describe the time-invariant ex-planatory variables, such as proxies for health status, income, and prices, that were used in these models.

[11] Specific questions and answers used to create the dietary knowledge score are available from the authors upon request.

[12] We chose this technique over creating a similar dichotomous variable because some eating occasions contain foods from multiple sources.

[13] The share of calories consumed away from home may also be correlated with the time-specific error term. We had originally treated this variable as endogenous, but the resulting in-strumental variable (IV) estimator was overidentified. We chose to focus on the endogeneity involved with the interval between meals because of our theoreti-cal model.

[14] This requires us to drop the fi rst eating occasion of each day.

[15] One alternative adopted by both Park and Davis (2001) and Abdulai and Aubert (2004) is to follow the method developed by Lewbel (1997), where the second and third moments of the endogenous variables are used as additional instruments in the IV estimation. We pursued this strategy as well, but found that in all cases, the models were overidentifi ed.

[16] For all simulations, we assume the respondent scores 75 on the knowledge index, works 40 hours per week, has gone 4 hours between meals, and eats all of his or her foods at home. We use mean values for meal name and weekend. We then change each assumption to estimate the effect of changing values of interest.

In: Maintaining a Healthy Diet
Editor: Anna R. Bernstein

ISBN: 978-1-60741-856-6

Chapter 2

COULD BEHAVIORAL ECONOMICS HELP IMPROVE DIET QUALITY FOR NUTRITION ASSISTANCE PROGRAM PARTICIPANTS?

United States Department of Agriculture

ABSTRACT

Findings from behavioral and psychological studies indicate that people regularly and predictably behave in ways that contradict some standard assumptions of economic analysis. Recognizing that consumption choices are determined by factors other than prices, income, and information illuminates a broad array of strategies to influence consumers' food choices. These strategies expand the list of possible ideas for improving the diet quality and health of participants in the U.S. Department of Agricul-ture's (USDA) Food Stamp Program; the Special Supplemental Nutrition Program for Women, Infants, and Children (WIC); and the National School Lunch and School Breakfast Programs.

Keywords: behavioral economics, food consumption, obesity, food stamps, National School Lunch Program, nutrition assistance, WIC

ACKNOWLEDGMENTS

The authors greatly appreciate the thoughtful review suggestions from Joanne Guthrie and Elizabeth Frazao, Economic Research Service (ERS); Marianne Bertrand, Univer-sity of Chicago; Steve Carlson, Rich Lucas, and Carol Olander, Food and Nutrition Service (FNS); Sean Cash, University of Alberta; and Trent Smith, Washington State University. We also thank Priscilla Smith for editorial and production assistance and Victor B. Phillips, Jr., for cover design and layout.

SUMMARY

As obesity has come to the forefront of public health concerns, there is growing interest in finding ways to guide consumers' food choices to be more beneficial for their long-term health. About one in five Americans participates in at least one of the nutrition assistance programs sponsored by the U.S. Department of Agriculture. This study uses behavioral economics, food marketing, and psychology to identify possible options for improving the diets and health of participants in the Food Stamp Program; the Special Supplemental Nutrition Program for Women, Infants, and Children (WIC); and the National School Lunch and School Breakfast Programs.

What Is the Issue?

USDA and other public health agencies historically have provided recom-mendations on how to make food choices that promote health and prevent disease. Food manufacturers and marketers, on the other hand, have discov-ered that certain psychological cues, such as packaging and presentation, are efficient ways to increase consumption of their products. Could similar marketing approaches be used in public health efforts to improve diet quality and reduce body weight among U.S. food assistance program partic-ipants? Insights from behavioral economics shed light on several factors that could help economists and policymakers better understand food choices. In 2005, over half of all nutrition assistance program participants were chil-dren. Many notions about what is good or acceptable to eat are determined in childhood. Improving diet quality among these nutrition program partici-pants has the potential to guide food choices at a critical time, when a child's dietary preferences are being defined.

What Did the Study Find?

This study incorporates findings from behavioral economics, food marketing, and psychology to propose insights into how people make food decisions. Recognizing that consumption choices are determined by factors other than prices, income, and information broadens the array of strategies that could influ-ence consumer food choices and improve diet and health. This exploration of new ideas, however, is by no means a recommendation or endorsement of any of them. A thorough analysis of costs, benefits, and potential impacts would be needed before any strategy could be considered as a policy option.

People have problems of self-control when choosing food, either because they prefer immediate gratification or because they are under the influence of a visceral factor, such as feeling hungry. Allowing them to preselect more healthful choices may be effective. For example, letting students preselect menu options in the National School Lunch or School Breakfast Programs or giving food stamp participants the option to preorder groceries by tele-phone or online may improve the healthfulness of their food choices.

People place more weight on "default options." Another idiosyncrasy of consumer choice frequently observed in experimental studies is that individ-uals exhibit an asymmetry in how they value gains relative to losses. This asymmetry gives rise to anomalous behavior, where individuals are willing to pay much less to acquire an item than they are willing to accept to part with it. It also makes them much more likely to choose the default options, even when the costs of switching to an alternative are low or even zero. Making the default menu option of school meals more healthful, such as a fruit salad instead of French fries may increase the likelihood that they will choose more healthful foods.

People categorize income into mental accounts. "Mental accounting" helps explain why coupons that can be used only for food purchases have been shown to be more effective at raising food spending among food stamp participants than an equal benefit amount of cash. If funds are earmarked for a specific purpose, recipients spend within a certain category until funds are entirely depleted. Specifying amounts of food stamp allotments that go toward the purchase of healthful foods, such as fruits, dark green vegetables, and whole grains, may be another option for improving diet quality of program participants.

People undervalue fixed costs relative to variable costs. When only certain items can be selected using prepayment (fixed costs), those items will be chosen more often than those that can be purchased only with cash (variable costs). In the school meals programs, for instance, students, in conjunction with parents or guardians, could specify that only more healthful items be purchased with prepaid cards.

Food decisions are often based more on emotion than rational thought. Impulsive behavior, such as choosing less healthy foods over healthier foods, may result from how the food is presented, the presence of stress, or other demands on an individual's "processing" ability. When processing resources are low, it is more likely that an individual will make consumption choices based solely on immediate considerations. Drawing attention to more healthful foods—by making them more accessible or displaying them more prominently in school cafeterias—might mitigate the effects of a distracting environment and increase the likelihood that students choose more healthful menu options.

External cues can have a major effect on the food selected, the amount consumed, and the eater's perception of how much was consumed. Noise levels, lighting, and distractions, as well as the size and shape of foods and food containers, affect how much people eat. Adjusting these factors can have a major impact on how much is eaten for a meal or snack. Reducing the number of students seated at each table or making school cafeterias more brightly lit are possible options that might help students better monitor their actual consumption.

How Was the Study Conducted?

This study incorporates findings from behavioral economics, food marketing, and psychology to explore various methods of improving individuals' diets and health. Within the context of USDA nutrition assistance programs, such as food stamps, WIC, and the school meals programs, these findings provide an oppor-tunity to begin thinking of new ways to encourage program participants to choose diets that are better aligned with their own goals for future health.

INTRODUCTION

USDA and other public health agencies have a long history of disseminating information about why and how to make food choices that promote health and prevent disease. Since 1980, recommendations on attaining adequate nutrition also include information about the benefits of maintaining a healthy body weight and limiting consumption of nutrients linked to chronic diseases. On the other side of the table, food manufacturers and marketers have discovered that certain psychological cues, such as packaging and presentation, are efficient ways to increase consumption of their products. These approaches have not been widely used in public health efforts aimed at improving diet quality and reducing body weight.

There are several behavioral and cognitive biases affecting food consumption decisions. The food psychology literature has found that external cues can drastically alter not only consumption volume, but also individual perceptions of how much they should and actually do eat. Wansink (1996) finds that larger packages lead to greater consumption and Diliberti et al. (2004) find that by increasing restaurant portion sizes from 248 grams to 377 grams of pasta, individuals increase caloric intake by an average of 43 percent. Also, more standard elements that are thought to be the main drivers of food choices, such as price, will sometimes prove to have little influence over consumption volume. For example, individuals appear to consume much larger quantities of food when it is stockpiled regardless of the initial cost (Wansink and Deshpande, 1994).

As obesity has come to the forefront of public health concerns, there is growing interest in finding ways to guide consumers' food choices to be more beneficial for their long-term health. One frequently mentioned option, the "snack tax," would raise the relative price of less healthful foods. However, taxes on food would disproportionately burden low-income indi-viduals who spend a greater share of their income on food than wealthier consumers. Also, such measures would impose an additional cost for everyone, not just consumers who need incentives to better balance their own long-term health preferences with current food choices. Thus, a major challenge is to find incentives that can improve the food choices among individuals who behave contrary to their own intentions without limiting the choices of individuals who make optimal choices.

A benefit of incorporating findings from food psychology and behavioral economics into this discussion is that it broadens the policy options. Food psychology research shows that subtle incentives, such as product placement, package size, and fixed-cost pricing (e.g., “all you can eat” buffets) used to increase consumption should be just as effective at reducing consumption. Moreover, review of the literature suggests that these tools may be at least as powerful as the more traditional economics tools used to guide consumers’ decisions, such as taxes and credits. And, unlike taxes or credits, behavioral cues can provide benefits to society without imposing a cost to those who currently behave optimally for their own long-term benefit, nor will they necessarily impose additional costs to those who are food insecure or living at the margins. However, a thorough analysis of costs, benefits, and potential impacts—a task outside the scope of this discussion—would be needed before any strategy proposed in this report could be considered a viable option.

Standard economic analysis relies primarily on large-scale survey data. By contrast, the field of behavioral economics typically tests hypotheses through the use of experiments that isolate behaviors—for example, the effect of larger portion sizes on a person’s food consumption. Typically the behavior of a group receiving the treatment of interest is compared with the behavior of a control group not receiving the treatment. In this case, consumption volume would be compared between those who were given the larger portions and those who were not. By randomly assigning individuals to either control or treatment groups, researchers can account for many confounding factors, such as selection biases. In this example, a selection bias may arise if hungry individuals choose both to give themselves larger portions and eat more as well. Without randomly assigning portion sizes, researchers would overestimate the effect of portion size on consumption. These methods can reveal more nuanced information than standard techniques, while also reducing the potential for confounding effects to mislead researchers.

This study’s objective is to incorporate the findings from behavioral economics, food marketing, and psychology into a framework that can be used to explore new methods of improving individuals’ diets and health. Beyond nutrition guidance and food labeling, few policies influence the food choices of the general population. However, there are mechanisms that directly influence the diets of those Americans who receive nutrition assistance. USDA’s domestic nutrition assistance programs affect the daily lives of millions of people. About one in five Americans participates in at least one nutrition assistance program at some point during the year. Many of these programs include nutrition education components and are designed to support healthy food choices. However, these individuals are more at risk than others from changes in the economy or other social conditions, including increased risk of diet-related illness (Fox and Cole, 2004). Finding additional ways to improve the healthfulness of food choices among this population without imposing additional costs or restricting their right to choose the foods they like as part of their nutrition assistance program participation could have broad societal benefits.

In 2005, more than half of the people who participated in either the Food Stamp Program or the Special Supplemental Nutrition Program for Women, Infants, and Children were children (Barrett, 2006; Oliveira, 2006). On average, over 29 million children participated in the National School Lunch Program each day (USDA, Food and Nutrition Service, 2006). Many of the notions about what is good or acceptable to eat are determined in the first few years of life (Smith, 2004), and people form their diets based on what foods are more familiar (Smith, 2004; Smith and Tasnadi, 2007). Thus, finding ways to improve diet quality among those participating in nutrition assistance programs is also important because these programs have the potential to guide food choices at a critical time—when a child's dietary preferences are being defined.

This study focuses on four of the largest nutrition assistance programs: the Food Stamp Program; the Special Supplemental Nutrition Program for Women, Infants, and Children; and the National School Lunch and Breakfast Programs, referred to collectively as USDA school meals programs (see the ERS *Food Assistance Landscape* series for details of each program; the most recent *Landscape* is available at http://www.ers.usda.gov/publications/ eib6-4). The potential for impact on food choices within the food stamp, WIC, and USDA school meals programs differs significantly depending on the nutrition assistance delivery mechanism. WIC and the FSP provide assistance for individuals to purchase food to be prepared and eaten within the home. The school meals programs offer prepared meals to be eaten within a school-controlled cafeteria. WIC provides for a very narrow set of products, while the FSP performs much like a direct money transfer, barring only nonfood items and prepared foods that are not intended for home consumption.

While the potential to exploit certain idiosyncratic behaviors to encourage healthier diets exists in all of these programs, the potential instruments differ substantially. Which interventions are viable will depend largely on whether a program distributes benefits by providing purchasing power or preparing meals. Bestowing benefits through prepared meals offers a great degree of control over both how the food is presented and the environment where the food is chosen. Manipulation of food to be prepared and eaten at home may be much more invasive or costly and may therefore require exploiting a very different set of behaviors.

PRICES, INCOME, AND INFORMATION ARE STANDARD POLICY LEVERS THAT INFLUENCE FOOD CHOICE

The standard economic framework for evaluating consumer behavior treats food as a good that provides both short- and long-term benefits. While some aspects of food, such as flavor, texture, and relief from hunger provide immediate gratification, the effect of other aspects, such as nutrient content, calories, and the presence of certain bacteria, are not usually realized until some point in the future. In line with the saying, "a moment on the lips, a lifetime on the hips," economic analysis of food choices typically assumes that individuals must make tradeoffs between enjoyment of today's choices and the consequences of those choices at some point in the future. How well individuals are able to translate food choices into future health outcomes is related to how much they know about diet, health, and nutrition.

Typically, this framework is then used to evaluate if and how much food choices will vary with three primary economic variables: income, prices, and information about diet and health. Historically, providing information about diet and health has been the most widely used tool to help consumers make more healthful food choices. For over 100 years, USDA has provided advice on how and why to eat a healthful diet (Welsh, Davis, and Shaw, 1993). Since 1980, USDA and the U.S. Department of Health and Human Services have jointly issued the *Dietary Guidelines for Americans* every 5 years. Although there have been variations over time, the primary focus has been on educating consumers in ways to achieve proper nutrition while consuming reasonable proportions of the various food groups in moderation.

In 1990, Congress passed the Nutrition Labeling and Education Act (NLEA), which requires that all packaged foods have nutrition labeling and use standardized definitions for terms such as serving size, "low fat," and "light." Many of the government-funded food and nutrition programs, such as food stamps, WIC, and the school meals programs, also earmark funds for nutrition education. The evidence is mixed on whether information and labels actually improve the healthfulness of food choices. Several studies have found a positive correlation between nutrition knowledge and diet quality, such as lower fat intake (Gould and Lin, 1994), the probability of being obese (Nayga, 2000b; Variyam and Cawley, 2006), and food label use (Nayga, 2000a). Others, however, have found no significant correlation or one that may be very short-lived (e.g., Chang and Just, 2007).

Rising obesity rates have led some health researchers to advocate raising the price of less healthful foods, such as salty snack chips, soft drinks, and ice cream, relative to more healthful foods, such as fruits, vegetables, and whole grains. Logistical problems aside, economic analysis of consumer's sensitivity to prices shows that such a measure would have limited efficacy because peoples' diets are not very responsive to prices. Using 1999 scanner data on food purchases, Kuchler, Tegene, and Harris (2005) estimate that taxing potato chips by 20 percent would bring about only a quarter-pound loss in body weight per year per potato-chip eater. Changing prices could also have some unintended consequences due to the interdependent nature of food choices. Kinsey and Bowland (1999) found that modest decreases in the price of fruits, meats, and dairy products would lead to small improvements in individuals' diet quality and that the price of fat would have to rise by as much as 15 percent to bring about a 1-percent reduction in fat consumption. Huang (1999) estimated that changing prices would also lead to some peculiar substitutions—decreasing the price of fruits or vegetables would increase consumption of fat, decreasing the price of vegetables would decrease consumption of vitamin A, and increasing the price of fat would reduce consumption of protein, calcium, iron, and folate. Such research shows that simply manipulating food prices is not likely to induce significant improvements in American consumers' diets.

The full "price" of food also includes the value of time spent acquiring, preparing, cooking, and cleaning up after meals. Many of the market-driven changes to the current U.S. food distribution system have reduced the time required to procure and prepare food by providing convenient, ready-to-eat snack foods, microwavable meals, vending machines at workplaces and schools, and drive-through windows at fast-food restaurants. These changes may have inadvertently made the environment more fat-friendly for consumers. It is extremely easy to access large quantities of food and expend hardly any time or energy doing so.

There is evidence that an increased availability of convenient foods is one underlying cause of increased consumption. This explanation conforms with standard economic theory, which predicts that people will consume more of an item whose total cost (combination of time and money) of production has declined (Cutler, Glaeser and Shapiro, 2003; Variyam, 2005). Cutler, Glaeser, and Shapiro (2003) found that prices, income, calorie expenditures (exercise), and caloric intake at meals all remained relatively stable during the period that obesity rates began increasing. The amount of time spent preparing food dropped by about 50 percent, thus the time cost of a snack declined sharply. Chou, Grossman, and Saffer (2004) also examine the effects of monetary prices and convenience (via an increased availability of fast food and other food sources) on obesity levels. While the relationship between food prices and obesity is statistically significant, it is small in magnitude. Availability of fast food, on the other hand, appears to play a much larger role in obesity. This indicates that while Americans may not be so responsive to monetary costs of food, they may be more sensitive to time costs.

This brief overview illuminates how a fairly standard economic framework can help explain some of the reasons behind food choices, but that the impact of standard economic levers—and the policy options associated with them—are limited. The next sections show that adding more realism into economic models by incorporating the psychological and behavioral aspects of food consumption reveals a broader range of policy options to increase the likelihood that individuals will make more healthful food choices.

How Cognitive Glitches and Psychological Biases Influence What People Eat

Through carefully controlled experiments, psychologists and behavioral researchers have documented widespread observance of behaviors and problem-solving techniques that do not conform with standard assumptions of standard economic theory. For example, experiments where subjects are asked to perform fairly simple reasoning tasks, such as calculating the prob-ability that event A will occur given event B, show that the vast majority of respondents make systematic errors. Psychologists infer that these errors are the result of individuals' using simple decision rules, or heuristics, which lead to seemingly illogical choices or biases (Conlisk, 1996; Kahneman, Slovic, and Tversky, 1982). These errors become more prevalent when deci-sions are made when there is some element of chance or uncertainty about the results of a choice or when some rewards from a decision are realized after a significant passage of time, rather than immediately. While using simple heuristics may lead to biases, doing so may still be a more efficient approach to problem solving if it provides an adequate solution without the greater time and mental costs of a more deliberative approach. Experimental research findings suggest that the heuristics used to simplify decisionmaking can predictably affect which foods they eat, how much, and their willing-ness to consume that food again. Experimental and theoretical research also describes how problems of self-control may arise when the benefits from a decision are separated from the costs by a time lag.

Making Changes, by Default

One idiosyncrasy of consumer choice frequently observed in experimental studies is that individuals exhibit an asymmetry in how they value gains relative to losses. Known as loss aversion (Kahneman and Tversky, 1984), this asymmetry gives rise to anomalous behavior, known either as an endowment effect (Thaler, 1980) or a status quo bias (Samuelson and Zeck-hauser, 1988). Both anomalies refer to aversions that cause individuals to willingly pay much less to acquire an item than they would accept to part with it (Samuelson and Zeckhauser, 1988; Kahneman, Knetsch, and Thaler, 1990). This aversion also makes individuals much more likely to choose the default options, even when the costs of switching to a different option are low (or even negative). For example, Choi et al. (2003) found that only 26 percent to 69 percent of employees opted to participate in a 401(k) program when they were not automatically enrolled compared with participation rates of 85 percent among employees for whom the default option was to enroll. Similarly, Thaler and Benartzi (2004) found that saving rates increased dramatically when employees were offered a plan where a specified fraction of their future pay increases were automatically diverted into a savings account.

Such findings from behavioral experiments suggest that individuals will be apt to make decisions that are more harmonious with their long-term objectives when those decisions are presented as the default options. Relating this to USDA's nutrition assistance programs, one way to increase the likelihood that program participants make healthier food choices would be to make such choices the default. Within the school cafeteria framework, a healthy meal could be automatically preordered for students each day. Students who wanted a different, less healthful food choice (such as a la carte offerings) would then have to change their order and pay the cost difference, if any. Among Food Stamp Program participants, the default option could be a more restrictive food stamp package that fulfilled certain nutrition guidelines, such as a minimum percentage of the benefit amount to be allocated to purchase of whole-grain foods, dark green vegetables, or fruits. To opt out of this package, participants would need to specify that they would prefer the current benefit program.

The characteristics of the goods or services in question as utilitarian or hedonic have been found to play a role in how likely individuals are to exhibit status quo biases. Hedonic characteristics are associated with a sensory experience and immediate gratification. Utilitarian attributes, on the other hand, are more functional and typically associated with a longer term goal, such as good health (Hirshman and Holbrook, 1982; Strahilevitz and Myers, 1998). Individuals tend to view goods in terms of moral structure— classifying them as "wants" or "shoulds" (Bazerman, Tenbrunsel, and Wade-Benzoni, 1998). The notion that some goods are virtuous or necessary while others are sinful or extravagant leads to very different choice behavior. Dhar and Wertenbroch (2000) show that utilitarian characteristics are more important when deciding which goods to acquire and hedonic characteristics are more important in determining which to give up. Thus, while individuals appear to be deliberative in determining which products to select, they seem to be more reactionary when choosing which items to forgo.

In the context of food, this suggests that individuals are more likely to add utilitarian foods (which are likely to be healthier) to their diet than they are to eliminate a hedonic (and typically less healthful) food. This odd twist on the status quo bias works against efforts to reduce consumption of foods that are viewed as extravagant, making it much more difficult to reduce caloric intake. These findings also support the concept of considering the healthfulness of default menu items and food packages within the nutrition assistance programs.

Distractions, Cognition, and Eating

Certain situations also affect the likelihood that individuals' decisions will be based more on emotional than on rational factors. Epstein (1993) proposes the Cognitive-Experiential Self Theory (CEST) to describe this conflict. This model supposes that there are two processes used to evaluate every stimulus:

1. An experiential system to make rapid evaluations based on emotions.

2. A cognitive process to make more deliberative evaluations based on rational thinking.

The primary determinant of which process takes over is the availability of processing resources (time, necessity to deal with other decisions, etc.). Impulsive behavior, such as choosing less healthy foods over healthy foods, may result from the presentation of food choices, the presence of stress, or other demands on processing ability. Shiv and Fedorikhin (1999) find that individuals who were given some cognitive task to perform while choosing between cake or fruit salad were much more likely to choose the cake than those given only the food-choice task. This result held true even if the price of the cake was raised considerably higher than the price of the fruit salad.

The standard economic framework can be adjusted to incorporate the possibility that individuals toggle between using a cognitive process to make decisions and an experiential system to make decisions based primarily on emotions. If it is true that emotions take precedence over reason as processing resources decrease, then another way to improve the healthfulness of individuals' food choices is to manage their processing resources. When processing resources are low, it is more likely that an individual will make consumption choices based solely on immediate considerations. When these resources are higher, the same individual will be more likely to consider the tradeoffs between current consumption and future well-being.

Within the school meals programs, processing resources could be affected by distractions or time constraints that occur while making meal selections or choosing when to stop eating. Consequently, students may be more likely to make healthful menu selections or more reasonable quantity decisions if afforded more time in which to do so. Alternatively, the nutritional value of foods chosen might improve if individuals were given the opportunity to make selections in a calmer environment—possibly in class, before heading to the cafeteria. Another way to mitigate the effect of a distracting environment would be to draw attention to the more healthful foods by making them more accessible or displaying them more prominently. Within the FSP or WIC, processing resources might again correspond to similar distractions or time constraints. A possible way to mitigate these factors would be to give participants the option of preselection or preordering their grocery items (whether program-provided or not) at times when fewer distractions might be present.

Mental Accounting

Lowering the price of one good, food for example, will have both an income and a substitution effect, according to standard economic predictions. With the income effect, individuals increase food purchases in response to more room in their budget. This change in price may also have a substitution effect, where people change how they allocate expenditures among broad categories. In this case, lowering food prices may lead to only a slight increase in total food purchases while generating a much greater increase in expenditures on other items.

By contrast, mental accounting (Thaler, 1980; Shefrin and Thaler, 2004) supposes that individuals categorize their income by earmarking it for specific purposes or specifying that it be used within a certain timeframe. The idea that money is not fungible but is set aside for a specific purpose is engrained in consumers' vocabularies early on with terms such as "lunch money," "rainy day funds," and "mad money." Income sources seen as one-time events are viewed as more frivolous (such as tax refunds) and are subsequently earmarked for more frivolous consumption (like plasma televisions). Individuals may also categorize a certain amount of income for food consumption based on factors such as the source of income (employment, welfare, food stamps, and gifts).

In contrast to the more standard framework, mental accounting predicts that once money is earmarked for a purpose, one will spend within a certain category until funds are entirely depleted. Thus, if allocating a portion of income to current food spending, and food prices decline, one may overlook the opportunity to shift the surplus "food money" to another purpose. Instead, one will buy more food. In this case, finding a low price on an item may lead to overconsumption rather than substitution.

Another consequence of mental accounting is that individuals tend to exhibit a "flat-rate bias," where they undervalue fixed costs, relative to variable costs (Thaler, 2004). Health club members typically choose to pay for their gym membership on a monthly or annual basis, even when a per-use fee would have lower total costs (DellaVigna and Malmendier, 2002).[1] One implication of a flat-rate bias is that, when only certain items can be selected using prepayment, those items will be chosen with greater frequency compared with those that can be purchased only with cash.

The idea of earmarking funds and mental accounts may partially explain why several studies have found that food stamp coupons that can be used only for food purchases are more effective at raising food expenditures than an equal benefit amount given as cash even when both coupons and cash are used on food (reviewed in Fox, Hamilton, and Lin, 2004). This outcome is contrary to rational economic theory, which predicts that cash and coupons would have the same effect. This concept also lends support to the idea that providing further guidelines on the proportion of food stamp allotments that should go toward the purchase of healthful foods, such as fruits, dark green vegetables, and whole grains, could increase the purchase of more healthful items among program participants.

Foods that are part of the official USDA school meals must meet dietary standards. But, similar standards could also be placed on a la carte foods and foods sold separately from USDA school meals. Through prepaid cards, or point-of-sale (POS) technology, students, possibly in conjunction with parents, could specify what portion of their total bill should be spent on fruits, vegetables, desserts, or high-calorie beverages. Such options have already been tried in several school districts. The finding that individuals undervalue fixed costs relative to variable costs has possible implications for the school meals programs as well. To take advantage of this flat-rate bias, parents or students could prepay for specific, more healthful items. Other, less healthful items, such as soft drinks or high-fat desserts, could be purchased, but only with cash.[2]

Problems of Self-Control and Visceral Influences

Economic models typically assume individuals discount future utility exponentially, meaning that the value people place on future well-being is less than the value of today's well-being and the value of each subsequent time period decreases at a constant rate. However, experimental and empirical studies provide examples showing that actual consumer behavior cannot be reconciled with the assumption of exponential discounting. One frequently observed anomaly is that individuals often change how they rank a less preferable, yet more immediate reward relative to a preferable but delayed reward when the time delay between receiving either reward is changed equally (discussed by Laibson, 2004). A common example cited in the literature on experimental economics describes an individual who prefers one apple right now to two apples 24 hours from now, yet also prefers two apples in 51 days to one apple in 50 days (Thaler, 1981). Such time-inconsistent preferences find expression as a self-control problem, where one places extra value on more immediate rewards within the near term. This behavior has been linked to consistent shortfalls in retirement savings, and the need for penalties on early withdrawals of those savings (Laibson et al., 1998; Angeletos et al., 2001). In the case of food consumption, the would-be dieter may continually commit to cutting back on high-calorie foods after one more doughnut.

Repeated observation of time-inconsistent preferences has led some researchers to change this assumption by using a framework where decisionmakers lack self-control and choose alternatives that are usually less desirable or valuable over some timeframe simply because they are available sooner (see Gul and Pesendorfer, 2004, for a review). This adjustment to the more standard economic framework has been used to show that individuals can improve their longrun well-being through some sort of commitment mechanism that will enforce time consistency and set limits on current consumption levels (e.g., a 401(k) plan). Such curbs on one's ability to choose could never be a valuable tool if individuals had an ability to choose the best option after the fact.

Kivetz and Simonson (2002) found that individuals tended to choose luxury items as program rewards rather than the cash equivalent (or greater) because they feared lack of self-control would cause them to use the money for everyday expenses, and therefore, preclude their ability to afford the luxury item. This framework has also been used to explain a number of seemingly inconsistent preferences including: why individuals choose rela-tively more expensive annual gym memberships over "pay as you go" options, even though the latter would be less expensive for most users (DellaVigna and Malmendier, 2002); why problems of self-control coupled with decreasing time and monetary costs of food attainment may explain an increasing rise in obesity rates (Culter, Glaeser, and Shapiro, 2003); and why food stamp recipients reduce caloric intake as the days after food stamp receipt increase (Shapiro, 2005).

A limitation of such models, however, is that time-inconsistent behavior is attributed entirely to how soon a choice is available relative to its alterna-tives (Frederick, Loewenstein, and O'Donoghue, 2004; Loewenstein, 2004). In terms of food consumption, this means an individual will always be expected to choose the more immediately available food, regardless of his or her level of hunger. In reviewing the literature on weight loss, Herman and Polivy (2003) show that simply making some foods immediately available is not sufficient to induce binge eating.

To account for this, researchers have developed an alternate framework that allows a broader range of situations to trigger present biased behaviors (such as a self-control problem) by adding the assumption that certain visceral influences, such as feeling hunger, thirst, or pain, can add to or detract from how much enjoyment an individual gets from current consumption (Loewenstein, 2004). For example, a plate of nachos is not terribly enjoyable after a full meal. But these same nachos may seem extremely palatable to a hungry person. Also, a hungry person is likely to make short-sighted tradeoffs between immediate and delayed food, even if that person will be feeling just as hungry tomorrow.

This visceral factors framework differs from Cognitive-Experiential Self Theory (described earlier) which assumes that the availability of processing resources—related to factors such as the amount of time afforded to make a decision, level of stress, or presence of other distraction—dictates whether an individual takes a rational approach to decisionmaking or makes evalua-tions based on emotions. In comparison, the visceral factors framework assumes that while an individual uses rational thinking to evaluate decisions, the amount of utility derived from consuming a specific amount of some good—say, food—will change depending on the intensity of relevant visceral influences, such as feeling hungry, nervous, or nauseous.

For explaining food choices, the visceral factors framework can illuminate how and why certain situations give rise to time-inconsistent choices. In a more neutral state, an individual may choose to consume the types and quantities of foods that are consistent with his or her long-term health objectives. As visceral factors intensify, however, the perceived value of one's current well-being increases relative to the value of one's future well-being. Thus, consumption of goods that provide immediate gratification will be consumed in greater amounts compared with situations when visceral factors are less intense.

Using this framework, Mancino (2003) and Mancino and Kinsey (2004) show that hunger can lead to unhealthy choices, especially when combined with time constraints. As individuals become busier (and time constraints begin to tighten), more convenient food becomes a substitute for leisure time. Also, as individuals become busier, they may eat less often, allowing their feeling of hunger to get out of control, leading to overconsumption. This research suggests that busier lifestyles may have created an atmosphere where increasing the interval between meals leads individuals to periodically ignore health information, causing an increase in obesity.

The empirical evidence that individuals tend to lack self-control, either because they simply prefer immediate gratification or because they are under the influence of a visceral factor, suggests that allowing them to pre-select or commit to more healthful choices would be an effective means to counteract their tendency to make shortsighted, less healthful choices. Within the school meals programs, students will be more likely to choose foods that promote better health over those that simply provide immediate gratification if they choose their foods well before meal time. Alternatively, parents or children could devise a commitment mechanism, such as making certain foods off-limits. Through point-of-sale technologies, such mecha-nisms are currently increasing in popularity. Some schools employ POS systems through which parents can track what menu items their children purchase at school and even specify that their POS card preclude the purchase of specific items, such as soft drinks or high-fat desserts.

Similarly, within the Food Stamp Program (FSP), participants may be more likely to choose foods that are in sync with their long-term health objectives if they make their purchasing decisions before going to the store and finding themselves tempted with less healthful food options, such as salty snack chips, high-fat dessert products, and soft drinks. One way to do this would be through preordering. Another option would be to allow FSP participants to specify that certain less healthful foods be ineligible for purchase with their electronic benefit transfer (EBT) cards. A simpler, less costly alterna-tive currently used by some States as part of their Food Stamp and Nutrition Education programs would be to design curriculum that highlights the importance of planning meals, preparing shopping lists, and not shopping for groceries on an empty stomach or accompanied by children (Philips et al., 2000).

The monthly schedule for distributing food stamps has been cited as a potential cause of weight gain among participants. Because benefits are distributed only once a month, there is evidence of a period of overcon-sumption shortly after benefits are distributed, followed by a period of rationing, or under-consumption later in the cycle (Wilde and Ranney, 2000). This cycle may be even more pronounced among individuals with self-control problems—they will likely spend too much for current consumption at the expense of future consumption. Increasing the frequency of benefit disbursements could also function as another commitment mecha-nism. Thus, decreasing the amount available for current consumption at each decision period, while leaving total payment amount unchanged, should also boost one's ability to make time-consistent decisions.

Avoiding Temptation

A fundamental tenet of rational behavior is the axiom of the independence of irrelevant alternatives. The axiom asserts that if a person prefers option A to option B, then he or she will continue to prefer A to B even if a third, irrelevant option C is available. Frequent observation of behavior that violates this principle suggests that modeling choices under an assumption of complete rationality will be too restrictive and result in erroneous predictions about behavior. Instead, individuals seem to exhibit a "context effect" where the rankings of alternatives depend on other options offered in a choice set, even when those options are never chosen (Camerer and Loewenstein, 2004). Gul and Pesendorfer (2001) propose that individuals have preferences over the presence of temptations: The value of choosing a salad rather than a hamburger will be lower when tempting items like chocolate cake also appear on the menu, even if the cake is not chosen. Because cognitively better choices may lose their appeal when more hedonic choices are presented, Gul and Pesendorfer argue that removing tempting options that are typically considered less desirable will unambiguously improve individual well-being.

Presenting individuals with tempting alternatives may also be problematic if their willpower (ability to self-regulate) is a depletable resource (Ozdenoren, Salant, and Silverman, 2006). Experiments show that an individual's ability to exercise willpower is lower if he or she has recently engaged in prior acts of self-restraint (Baumeister and Vohs, 2003). While individuals who have honed their skills at self-regulation may find effective ways to stick with their long-term objectives (Fishbach and Shah, 2006), less effective regulators will be better able to avert temptation by imposing additional costs (or benefits) on giving in to temptation (Fishbach and Trope, 2005).

Within the school meals setting, these findings suggest that simply presenting students with a broader array of unhealthful but flavorful foods can decrease the enjoyment they get from choosing more healthful foods. The findings also suggest that the likelihood of choosing healthful menu options decreases as the number of tempting, less healthful options increases. Another finding from this research is that giving individuals the option of precommitting to the more healthful option may improve well-being. As such, offering students the option to preselect healthful menu options could be another way to improve their food choices. Through preordering their groceries, either by phone or possibly online, FSP participants could also be given the option to preselect their foods directly through FSP.

How Cognitive Glitches and Psychological Biases Influence How Much People Eat

In addition to choosing the wrong mix of foods, many Americans simply eat too much food as well. According to ERS data on food consumption, the average daily calories available in the U.S. food supply increased by more than 500 calories per person between 1970 and 2004. Surprisingly, experimental studies find that choosing what to eat and choosing how much to eat may be controlled by separate psychological mechanisms. Environmental factors seem to have a stronger effect on the amount people eat than tastes and preferences (Wansink and Kim, 2004). In particular, the eating environ-ment (atmosphere, effort, social facilitation, and distractions) and the food environment (salience, structure, size, stockpiling, and shape) affect consumption volume by setting consumption norms (an indication of how much people should consume) and inhibiting monitoring accuracy. These subtle cues can have large impacts on consumption volume, often without the individual's being aware of their effect (see Wansink, 2004, for defini-tions of terms and complete review of the consumption volume literature).

Where We Eat and with Whom

The eating environment is defined as all factors external to the presentation of the food itself. Social situations may encourage individuals to eat more than they would normally. When eating in groups or social situations, individuals tend to eat quantities that are similar to others (Birch and Fisher, 2000; de Castro, 1994). Individuals may alter what they eat due to the distraction of conversation and increase consumption volume as the size of the gathering increases (de Castro and Brewer, 1992) or as the length of meal is extended (Bell and Pliner, 2003). When wanting to impress others at the table, as in a job interview, individuals will often eat less (Chaiken and Pliner, 1990; Mori, Chaiken, and Pliner, 1987, Stroebele and de Castro, 2004). Social gatherings also tend to decrease the variance of consumption; those who normally eat large amounts eat less, while those who normally eat little will eat more (Clendennen, Herman, and Polivy, 1994; Pliner et al., 2003).

Other aspects of the eating environment, such as lighting, odor, and temperature, can influence consumption volume (Wansink, 2006; Wansink, 2004). People tend to shorten the duration of meals in brightly lit environments compared with places that are more dimly lit. People also tend to be less self-conscious when the lighting is low, thus increasing the likelihood of eating more than they would normally.

Beyond mentioning their impact as part of nutrition education, it is difficult to imagine how controlling where people eat, with whom, or the atmosphere within a dining area could be feasible within either FSP or WIC. However, these findings do have implications within the school meals programs. It may be that simply decreasing the number of students seated at each table could have a significant impact on the amount of food consumed at school meals. Making school cafeterias more brightly lit could be another way to help students better monitor their actual consumption volume.

How Food Is Presented— Salience and Stockpiling

The primary factor in managing consumption volume is the accuracy with which individuals gauge how much they eat (Arkes, 1991; Polivy et al., 1986). Rules of thumb, such as eating one package or one bowlful of food or choosing products that are lower in fat or calories, are often used to monitor consumption volume. Such rules of thumb can have unintended effects on dieters. For example, Wansink and Linder (2003) found that while diners correctly believed that dipping bread in olive oil would increase the fat content relative to spreading butter on the bread, their total consumption volume may have negated this difference. These same diners tended to eat 23 percent more bread during the course of the meal when choosing butter over olive oil (Wansink and Linder, 2003).

Increasing the salience of food may increase consumption volume because it serves as a reminder of a pleasurable experience. Simply seeing a food can also lead to unplanned consumption (Boon et al., 1998; Cornell, Rodin, and Weingarten, 1989). Salience may be generated internally, leading to greater consumption volume than externally generated salience. Scientists were able to manipulate the salience of soup by simply asking individuals to write a description of the last time they ate soup. Those asked to describe their experience consumed more than twice as much soup in the next 2 weeks as did a control group that was not asked (Wansink and Deshpande, 1994).

Similarly, individuals who happened by a cookie dish, and impulsively decided to eat, ate fewer cookies than those who deliberately sought out the cookies (Wansink, 1994). Conversely, placing candies just 3 feet away from one's desk, as opposed to directly on one's desk, can significantly reduce the volume of consumption (by five to six chocolates a day, see Painter, Wansink and Heiggelke, 2002).

Stockpiling food can also increase consumption (Chandon and Wansink, 2002). In an experiment where homes were stocked with large quantities of ready-to-eat food, the foods were consumed at greater than twice the rate of consumption than in homes given more normal amounts of the food within the first week (Chandon and Wansink, 2002). After the first week, consumption rates were similar between the two treatments. Some have speculated that stockpiled foods may increase visibility and salience of the food. However, experiments attempting to isolate this phenomenon have been inconclusive (Terry and Beck, 1985; Wansink and Deshpande, 1994).

Devising ways to directly manipulate the salience of foods within the WIC or food stamp program is difficult to imagine. However, nutrition education within these programs could highlight ways to increase the salience of certain foods, such as fruits and vegetables, relative to other less healthful foods by changing where they are stored within the home. The school meals programs, on the other hand, have the ability to work with cafeterias and lunchrooms to change the placement of specific food items to adjust their relative prominence. Salads, fruit and vegetable servings, or other more healthful foods could be displayed more prominently, such as at the beginning of the cafeteria lines or on a level that is easily accessible. By contrast, desserts, soft drinks, or other less nutrient-dense foods could be offered so they are harder to reach and harder to see.

The finding that stockpiled foods are consumed in greater quantity may have implications for how benefits are distributed within the Food Stamp Program. There is speculation that the monthly food stamp benefit disbursement contributes to sporadic consumption of food. Shortly after benefits are issued, food expenditures spike and thus foods are more plentiful within the home compared with the end of the month.[3] If recently stockpiled foods are consumed in greater quantity, program participants, especially among those who have problems of self-control, would be more likely to experience binge-eating at the beginning of the food stamp cycle. Therefore, allowing FSP participants to choose to have benefits distributed more frequently could reduce the variation in the quantity (and possibly quality) of food intake throughout the month.

How Food Is Presented—Variety, Shape of Container, and Packaging

The structure or variety of food can also lead to increased consumption volume. In particular, offering a greater variety of foods increases the consumption volume of that food (Miller et al., 2000; Rolls, 1986; Rolls et al., 1981). Recent work has found that even increasing aspects of variety not associated with taste or nutrition significantly increases consumption volume. For example, subjects presented with 10 versus 7 colors of M&M candies consumed 43 percent more candy (Kahn and Wansink, 2004). Another experiment presented one set of subjects with identical numbers and variety of colors of jelly beans. However, while one treatment group received the jelly beans sorted by color, the other received the assortment mixed. Those who received the mixed assortment ate 69 percent more on average (Kahn and Wansink, 2004).

Larger portion sizes are frequently cited as contributors to increased obesity rates in the United States (Rolls, 2003; Young and Nestle, 2002). Experimental research does show that people eat more when presented with larger packages or portions of food (Diliberti et al., 2004; Rolls et al., 2004; Wansink, 1996; Nisbett, 1968; Rolls, Morris, and Roe, 2002; Edelman et al., 1986). Doubling the portion size increases consumption anywhere from 18 percent to 25 percent for meal-related foods and by up to 45 percent for snack foods (Wansink, 1996). Surprisingly, this result is robust to any number of different treatments. Larger portions lead to greater consumption even if the food is reported to be repulsive by the subjects (Wansink and Kim, 2004). Moreover, eating from larger packages causes less accuracy in monitoring consumption volume; when eating from larger packages, people underestimate their own consumption to a larger extent compared with when they eat from smaller packages (Wansink, 1996). Alternatively, increasing the calorie density appears to have little effect on consumption volume (Rolls, Bell, and Waugh, 2000; Rolls et al., 1998; Rolls, Morris, and Roe, 2002).

The shape of serving containers, such as bowls, plates and glasses, can also significantly affect the volume of consumption. Individuals tend to focus on the height of a glass rather than its width (Krider, Raghubir, and Krishna, 2001; Piaget, 1969; Raghubir and Krishna, 1999). Teenagers were found to pour 88 percent more juice into short, wide glasses than into tall, thin glasses, when both types of glasses held the same volume. Similarly, bartenders asked to pour 1.5 ounces of gin poured 26 percent more into tumbler-style glasses than into tall, thin glasses (Wansink and van Ittersum, 2003).

Lastly, there is evidence that other alterations in food packaging or presentation may make it easier to assess consumption volume. Introducing more intermediate packaging in containers of chips or other items, such as individually wrapped sets of cookies within a bag, seems to draw attention to consumption volume and make it easier for individuals to determine an appropriate stopping point (Wansink, 2004).

Compared with the FSP or WIC, it is more straightforward to apply implications from these findings to the school meals programs. Increasing the number of different vegetables or fruits offered within a single salad may lead students to consume a greater amount. Changing the shape of containers that are used could also promote consumption of certain foods and beverages relative to less healthful foods. Tall, thin glasses could be used for less healthful beverages while shorter, wider glasses could be used for beverages such as low-fat milk, water, and fruit juices. Similarly, larger bowls could be used for servings of fruits and vegetables, while small plates and dishes could be used for desserts or other less nutritious foods. Finally, placing packaging restrictions, such as 100-calorie packs, in vending machines and prepackaged foods a la carte is another way to help individuals monitor their own consumption volume within the schools.

In addition to highlighting the effects of variety, container shape, and product packaging on consumption volume in nutrition education for food stamp and WIC participants, there may be opportunities to apply some of the findings more directly. Interested program participants could be given a set of glasses, dishes, and/or bowls that contain some sort of visual graphic to indicate appropriate portion sizes. Promoting single-serving packaging for whole-grain cereals or low-fat cheese slices may also be feasible within the WIC package.

Psychological Biases Can Also Make People More Receptive to New Information

For some, improving diet quality may require eating different foods or changing methods of preparation. Experimental research finds that specific cues can significantly influence individuals' expectations of how a new product will taste and, thus, how likely individuals are to try new foods and recipes. These cues may include appearance, name, price, brand, or information and descriptions given by others (Tuorila et al., 1998; Cardello and Sawyer, 1992). Subsequently, expectations can bias an individual's actual postconsumption opinion of taste and overall experience. Experiments show that individuals who think an item will taste good give higher post-trial evaluations compared with those who expected the same item to taste bad (Tuorilla et al., 1998; Cardello and Sawyer, 1992).

Cardello and Sawyer (1992) told groups of subjects that they would be sampling a brand of juice from a new tropical fruit. Each group except one was told that the juice had been taste-tested previously and subjects had either "liked it very much," "disliked it very much," or "neither liked nor disliked it," depending on treatment group. Subjects' expectations about the juice correlated very closely with the information provided by the researchers. Groups whose members had expected a bad experience reported a lower level of acceptance than groups whose members had expected a good experience. This is a phenomenon called "confirmation." In fact, subjects' expectations about the overall experience tended to bias their post-trial analysis of taste sensations (like sweetness) that had not been mentioned in the pre-taste information. Despite biasing evaluations, it appears that discovering that food is not what was described reduces one's willingness to try the food again (Tuorila et al., 1998).

Individuals have been found to be significantly influenced by who gave them information about a product. Manufacturers and retailers have long known the power of word-of-mouth advertising. Smith (2004) also argues that many notions as to what is good or acceptable are determined in the first few years of life. This leads marketers of foods to frequently show images of young children who are happy presumably because they have consumed the marketers' food products.

People seek social validation by trying to fit in and are more likely to be persuaded by people they consider to be likable (Cialdini, 2001). Not surprisingly, that is why people who are considered popular and trustworthy figures are often used to tout the virtues of a product, rather than more infamous people. Promoters have now taken this one step further. It is now becoming increasingly popular among product promoters to actually seek out young adults or teenagers to act as "trend setters" who will be able to spread the word about a product among their peers (Walker, 2004).

In terms of providing nutrition education with school meals programs, FSP, and WIC, this suggests that who delivers the message and how satisfied he or she appears to be while doing so may have more of an impact than simply providing information about how and why to make more healthful food choices.

Conclusions

The previous sections summarized how the use of simple rules of thumb and heuristics may influence what individuals choose to eat, how much they eat, and how they evaluate these decisions after the fact. Incorporating these findings into the study of consumer behavior expands the array of possible ideas that may be considered for food policy, nutrition education, and social marketing.

With small adjustments, standard economic frameworks can incorporate more realism by recognizing that individuals often use simple heuristics, such as placing more weight on default options or using package size to determine quantity, when making food choices. The practical implications of this would be that altering elements of the product, such as package size and shape, the amount of variety, the number of calories, or the default options on a menu, can significantly affect diet quality and consumption volume.

Altering the food environment by increasing the convenience of healthful foods relative to less healthful foods, reducing distractions, or altering the lighting may also make it easier to make choices that are more harmonious with an individual's long-term health objectives.

Recognizing that situational cues, like hunger, stress, or distractions, can increase tendencies to focus on current well-being also expands possible policy and education techniques. Commitment devices, such as allowing individuals to preselect more healthful foods, may be another effective way to help indi-viduals make food choices that align with their own future health goals.

Similarly, explicitly modeling how mental accounting affects individuals' sensitivity to price differences reveals subtle techniques that might be able to significantly improve the quality of food choices. Knowing that people undervalue fixed costs relative to variable costs suggests that allowing people to prepay for healthful items may be another way to strengthen the link between intended and actual behavior.

Willingness to try new foods and a propensity to like them are strongly influenced by the actions of those around us. In terms of nutrition education and marketing, this suggests that who delivers the message and how satisfied they appear may have more of an impact than simple information about the virtues of healthful foods.

These findings expand the list of ideas for improving the diet quality among participants of specific food and nutrition programs, such as food stamps, WIC, and the school meals programs, without limiting freedom of choice. And unlike more traditional interventions, such as changing prices or banning specific food items, many of the proposed changes could be targeted to only those participants who wanted to make choices that are more harmonious with their own (or their parents') long-term health objectives.

This exploration of new ideas is by no means a recommendation or endorsement of any of them. A thorough analysis of costs, benefits, and potential impacts would be needed before any strategy could be considered as a policy option. Many of these suggested ideas may also influence where households shop, how they manage limited resources, and the total package of what they purchase. Practical and legal issues may also pose hurdles to implementing some of these strategies. As such, an important area for research would be to design experiments and pilot programs to gauge the efficacy, cost, legality, and feasibility of these possibilities. Comparing results of these experiments against estimated costs and benefits of more traditional approaches to nutrition assistance would also clarify the merits of these ideas relative to other strategies.

REFERENCES

Ainslie, G. & Haslam, N. (1992). "Hyperbolic Discounting" and "Self-Control," *Choice Over Time*, George Loewenstein and John Elster (eds.). New York: Russell Sage Foundation.

Angeletos, George-Marios, et al. (2001). "The Hyperbolic Consumption Model: Calibration, Simulation, and Empirical Evaluation." *Journal of Economic Perspectives*, *Vol. 15*, 47-68.

Akerlof, G. A. (1991). "Procrastination and Obedience." *American Economic Review*, *Vol. 81*, No. 2, 1-19.

Arkes, H. R. (1991). "Costs and Benefits of Judgment Errors–Implications for Debiasing." *Psychology Bulletin*, *Vol. 110*, 486-498.

Barrett, A. (2006). *Characteristics of Food Stamp Households: Fiscal Year 2005*. Report No. FSP-06-CHAR. Prepared by Mathematica Policy Research, Inc. for the U.S. Department of Agriculture, Food and Nutrition Service. Accessible at: www.fns.usda.gov/oane

Baumeister, Roy, and Kathleen Vohs. (2003). "Willpower, Choice, and Self-Control," *Time and Decision*, George Loewenstein, Daniel Read, and Roy Baumeister (ed.). New York: Russell Sage Foundation.

Bazerman, M. H., Tenbrunsel, A. E. & Wade-Benzoni, K. (1998). "Negotiating with Yourself and Losing: Understanding and Managing Conflicting Internal Preferences." *Academy of Management Review, Vol. 23*, 225-241.

Bell, R. & Pliner, P. L. (2003). "Time to Eat: The Relationship Between the Number of People Eating and Meal Duration in Three Lunch Settings." *Appetite*, *Vol. 41*, 215-218.

Birch, L. L. & Fisher, J. O. (2000). "Mother's Child-Feeding Practices Influence Daughters' Eating and Weight." *American Journal of Clinical Nutrition*, *Vol. 71*, 1,054-1,061.

Boon, B., Stroebe, W., Schut, H. & Jansen, A. (1998). "Food for Thought: Cognitive Regulation of Food Intake." *British Journal of Health Psychology*, *Vol. 3*, 27-40.

Bowman, D., Minehart, D. & Rabin, M. (1999). "Loss Aversion in a Consumption-Savings Model," *Journal of Economic Behavior and Organization*, *Vol. 38*, No. 2, 155-178(24).

Camerer, C. F. & Loewenstein, G. (2004). "Behavioral Economics: Past, Present and Future." *Advances in Behavioral Economics*, Colin F. Camerer, George Loewenstein, and Matthew Rabin (eds.). Russell Sage Foundation. Princeton, NJ: Princeton University Press, 3-52.

Cardello, A. V. & Sawyer, F. M. (1992). "Effects of Disconfirmed Consumer Expectations on Food Acceptability." *Journal of Sensory Studies*, *Vol. 7*, 253-277.

Chaiken, S. & Pliner, P. (1990). "Eating, Social Motives, and Self-Presentation in Women and Men." *Journal of Experimental Social Psychology*, *Vol. 26*, 240-254.

Chandon, P. & Wansink, B. (2002). "When Are Stockpiled Products Consumed Faster? A Convenience-Salience Framework of Postpurchase Consumption Incidence and Quantity." *Journal of Marketing Research*, *Vol. 39*, 321-335.

Chang, Hung-Hao, & David, R. Just. (2007). "Health Information Availability and the Consumption of Eggs: Are Consumers Bayesians?" *Journal of Agricultural and Resource Economics*, *Vol. 32*, No. 1, 77-92.

Choi, James, et al. (2003). "Optimal Defaults." *American Economic Review Papers and Proceedings*, May, 180-185.

Chou, Shin-Yi, Michael Grossman, and Henry Saffer. (2004). "An Economic Analysis of Adult Obesity: Results from the Behavioral Risk Factor Surveillance System." *Journal of Health Economics*, *Vol. 23*, No. 3, 565-587.

Cialdini, Robert. (2001). "The Science of Persuasion." *Scientific American*. February, 76-81.

Clendennen, V., Herman, C. P. & Polivy, J. (2003). "Social Facilitation of Eating Among Friends and Strangers." *Appetite*, *Vol. 23*, 1-13.

Cornell, C. E., Rodin, J. & Weingarten, H. (1989). "Stimulus-Induced Eating When Satiated." *Physiology and Behavior*, *Vol. 45*, 695-704.

Conlisk, John. (1996). "Why Bounded Rationality?" *Journal of Economic Literature*, *Vol. 34*, No. 2, 669-700.

Cutler, D. M., Glaeser, E. L. & Shapiro, J. M. (2003). "Why Have Americans Become More Obese?" *Journal of Economic Perspectives*, *Vol. 17*, 93-118.

de Castro, J. M. (1994). "Family and Friends Produce Greater Social Facilitation of Food Intake than Other Companions." *Physiology and Behavior*, *Vol. 56*, 445-455.

de Castro, J. M. & Brewer, E. (1992). "The Amount Eaten in Meals by Humans Is a Power Function of the Number of People Present." *Physiology and Behavior*, *Vol. 51*, 121-125.

DellaVigna, S. & Malmendier, U. (2002). *"Overestimating Self-Control: Evidence from the Health Club Industry" paper.* University of California, Berkley.

Dhar, R. & Wertenbroch, K. (2000). "Consumer Choice Between Hedonic and Utilitarian Goods." *Journal of Marketing Research*, *Vol. 37*, 60-71.

Diliberti, N., et al. (2004). "Increased Portion Size Leads to Increased Energy Intake in a Restaurant Meal." *Obesity Research*, *Vol. 12*, 562-568.

Edelman, B., Engell, D., Bronstein, P. & Hirsch, E. (1986). "Environmental Effects on the Intake of Overweight and Normal-Weight Men." *Appetite*, *Vol. 7*, 71-83.

Epstein, S. (1993). "Emotion and Self-Theory." *Handbook of Emotions*, In: M. Lewis, & J. M. Haviland (eds.). New York: Guilford, 313-326.

Fishbach, Ayelet, and James Shah. (2006). "Self-Control in Action: Implicit Dispositions Toward Goals and Away from Temptations." *Journal of Personality and Social Psychology*, *Vol. 90*, No. 5, 820-832.

Fishbach, Ayelet, and Yaacov Trope. (2005). "The Substitutability of External Control and Self-Control." *Journal of Experimental Social Psychology*, *Vol. 41*, 256-270.

Fox, Mary Kay, & Nancy Cole. (2004). *Nutrition and Health Characteristics of Low-Income Populations*. E-FAN-04014-1. U.S. Department of Agriculture, Economic Research Service. December.

Fox, Mary Kay, William Hamilton, and Biing-Hwan Lin (eds.). (2004). *Effects of Food Assistance and Nutrition Programs on Nutrition and Health: Volume 3, Literature Review.* Food Assistance and Nutrition Research Report No. 19-3, U.S. Department of Agriculture, Economic Research Service.

Frederick, Shane, George Loewenstein, and Ted O'Donoghue. (2004). "Time Discounting and Time Preference: A Critical Review." *Advances in Behavioral Economics*. Colin F. Camerer, George Loewenstein, and Matthew Rabin (eds.). Russell Sage Foundation. Princeton, NJ: Princeton University Press, pp.162-222.

Gould, B. W. & Lin, H. C. (1994). "Nutrition Information and Household Dietary Fat Intake." *Journal of Agricultural and Resource Economics* (19:2) December: 349-365.

Gul, Faruk, & Wolfgang Pesendorfer. (2001). "Temptation and Self-Control." *Econometrica, Vol. 69*, No. 6, 1,403-1,435.

Gul, Faruk, & Wolfgang Prosendorfer (2004). "Self-Control, Revealed Preference and Consumption Choice." *Review of Economic Dynamics, Vol. 7*, 243-264.

Herman, C. P. & Polivy, J. (2003). "Dieting As an Exercise in Behavioral Economics." *Time and Decision*. George Lowenstein, Daniel Reed, and Roy Baumeister (eds.). New York: Russell Sage Foundation, 459-489.

Hirschman, E. C. & Holbrook, M. B. (1982). "Hedonic Consumption: Emerging Concepts, Methods and Propositions." *Journal of Marketing, Vol. 46*, 92-101.

Huang, K. (1999). *Role of National Income and Prices in America's Eating Habits, Changes and Consequences*, E. Frazao (ed.). Agriculture Information Bulletin No. 750. U.S. Department of Agriculture, Economic Research Service.

Kahn, B. E. & Wansink, B. (2004). "The Influence of Assortment Structure on Perceived Variety and Consumption Quantities." *Journal of Consumer Research, Vol. 30*, 519-533.

Kahneman, D., Slovic, P. & Tversky, A. eds. (1982). *Judgement Under Uncertainty: Heuristics and Biases.* Cambridge: Cambridge University Press.

Kahneman, Daniel, & Amos Tversky. (1984). "Choices, Values, and Frames." *American Psychologist*, April, *Vol. 39*, 341-350.

Kahneman, D., Knetsch, J. L. & Thaler, R. H. (1990). "Experimental Tests of the Endowment Effect and the Coase Theorem." *Journal of Political Economy, Vol. 98*, 1,325-1,348.

Kahneman, D. & Tversky, A. (1991). "Loss Aversion in Riskless Choice: A Reference-Dependent Model." *Quarterly Journal of Economics*. Cambridge, MA: Harvard University, MIT Press.

Kinsey, J. & Bowland, B. (1999). "How Can the U.S. Food System Deliver Food Products Consistent With the Dietary Guidelines? Food Marketing and Retailing: An Economist's View." *Food Policy*, *Vol. 24*, 237-253.

Kivetz, R. & Simonson, I. (2002). "Earning the Right To Indulge: Effort As a Determinant of Customer Preference Toward Frequency Program Rewards." *Journal of Marketing Research*, *Vol. 39*, 155-170.

Krider, R. E., Raghubir, P. & Krishna, A. (2001). "Pizzas: or Square? Psychological Biases in Area Comparisons." *Marketing Science*, *Vol. 20*, 405-425.

Kuchler, Fred, Abebayehu Tegene, and Michael Harris. (2005). "Taxing Snack Foods: Manipulation Diet Quality or Financing Information Programs." *Review of Agricultural Economics*, *Vol. 27*, 4-20.

Laibson, David. (2004). "Golden Eggs and Hyperbolic Discounting." *Advances in Behavioral Economics*. Colin F. Camerer, George Loewenstein, and Matthew Rabin (eds.). Russell Sage Foundation. Princeton, NJ: Princeton University Press, 429-457.

Laibson, David, et al. (1998). "Self-Control and Saving for Retirement." *Brookings Papers on Economic Activity*, 91-196.

Loewenstein, George. (2004)."Out of Control: Visceral Influences on Behavior." *Advances in Behavioral Economics*. Colin F. Camerer, George Loewenstein, and Matthew Rabin (eds.). Russell Sage Foundation. Princeton, NJ: Princeton University Press, 689-724.

Mancino, Lisa. (2003). *Americans' Food Choices: The Interaction of Information, Intentions and Convenience*. Ph.D. dissertation. St. Paul: University of Minnesota, Department of Applied Economics.

Mancino, Lisa & Kinsey, Jean. (2004). "*Diet Quality and Calories Consumed: The Impact of Being Hungrier, Busier, and Eating Out.*" Working Paper 04-02, The Food Industry Center, University of Minnesota, St. Paul.

Miller, D. L., et al. (2000). "Effects of Dietary Fat, Nutrition Labels, and Repeated Consumption on Sensory-Specific Satiety." *Physiology and Behavior*, *Vol. 71*, 153-158.

Mori, D., Chaiken, S. & Pliner, P. (1987). "'Eating Lightly' and the Self-Presentation of Femininity." *Journal of Personality and Social Psychology*, *Vol. 53*, 693-702.

Mullainathan, Sendhil, & Richard H. Thaler. (2000). "*Behavioral Economics,*" National Bureau of Economic Research Working Paper 7948, National Bureau of Economic Research, Inc., Cambridge, MA.

Nayga, R. M. (2000a). "Nutrition Knowledge, Gender and Food Label Use." *Journal of Consumer Affairs*, *Vol. 34*, No. 1, Summer, 97-111.

Nayga, R. M. (2000b). "Schooling, Health Knowledge and Obesity." *Applied Economics*, *Vol. 32*, 815-822.

Nisbett, R. E. (1968). "Determinants of Food Intake in Human Obesity." *Science*, *Vol., 159*, 1,254-1,255.

O'Donoghue, Ted, & Matthew Rabin. (2004). "Doing It Now or Later." *Advances in Behavioral Economics.* Colin F. Camerer, George Loewenstein, and Matthew Rabin (eds.). Russell Sage Foundation. Princeton, NJ: Princeton University Press, 223-251.

Oliveira, Victor. (2006). *Food Assistance Landscape*, March 2006. Economic Information Bulletin 6-2, U.S. Department of Agriculture, Economic Research Service.

Ozdenoren, Emre, Stephen Salant, & Dan Silverman. (2006). "*Willpower and the Optimal Control of Visceral Urges*." National Bureau of Economic Research Working Paper 12278, National Bureau of Economic Research, Inc., Cambridge, MA.

Painter, J. E., Wansink, B. & Hieggelke, J. B. (2002). "How Visibility and Convenience Influence Candy Consumption." *Appetite*, *Vol. 38*, 237-238.

Phelps, E.S. & R. Pollak. (1968). "On Second-Best National Saving and Game-Equilibrium Growth." *Review of Economic Studies*. *Vol. 35*, 185-199.

Philips, Beverly, et al. (2000). "Money for Food: A Curriculum about Planning for and Spending Family Food Dollars. Wisconsin Education Program, available at www.uwex.edu/ces/wnep/teach/mff/mffall.pdf

Piaget, J. (1969). *The Mechanisms of Perception*. London, UK: Routledge & Kegan Paul.

Pliner, P., et al. (2003). "*Time To Eat? The Impact of Time Facilitation and Social Facilitation on Food Intake*." Presented at Pangborn Sensory Science Symposium, Boston, MA.

Polivy, J., et al. (1986). "The Effects of Self-Attention and Public Attention on Eating in Restrained and Unrestrained Subjects." *Journal of Personality and Social Psychology*. *Vol. 50*, 1,203-1,224.

Raghubir, P. & Krishna, A. (1999). "Vital Dimensions in Volume Perception: Can the Eye Fool the Stomach?" *Journal of Marketing Research*, *Vol. 36*, 313-326.

Rolls, B. J. (2003). "The Supersizing of America: Portion Size and the Obesity Epidemic." *Nutrition Today*, *Vol. 38*, 645-649.

Rolls, B. J., Bell, E. A. & Waugh, B. A. (2000). "Increasing the Volume of a Food by Incorporating Air Affects Satiety in Men." *American Journal of Clinical Nutrition*, *Vol. 72*, 361-368.

Rolls, B. J., et al. (1998). "Volume of Food Consumed Affects Satiety in Men." *American Journal of Clinical Nutrition*, *Vol. 67*, 1,170-1,177.

Rolls, B. J., Morris, E. L. & Roe. L. S. (2002). "Portion Size of Food Affects Energy Intake in Normal-Weight and Overweight Men and Women." *American Journal of Clinical Nutrition*, *Vol. 76*, 1,207-1,213.

Rolls, B. J., et al. (2004). "Increasing the Portion Size of a Packaged Snack Increases Energy Intake in Men and Women." *Appetite Vol. 42*, 63-69.

Rolls, B. J. (1986). "Sensory-Specific Satiety." *Nutrition Review*, *Vol. 44*, 93-101.

Rolls, B. J., et al. (1981). "Variety in a Meal Enhances Food Intake in Men." *Physiology and Behavior*, *Vol. 26*, 215-221.

Samuelson, William, and Richard Zeckhauser. (1988). "Status Quo Bias in Decision Making." *Journal of Risk and Uncertainty*, Springer, Netherlands, *Vol. 1*, No. 1, 7-59.

Shapiro, Jesse, M. (2005). "Is There a Daily Discount Rate? Evidence from the Food Stamp Nutrition Cycle." *Journal of Public Economics*, *Vol. 89*, 303-325.

Shefrin, Hersh, M. & Thaler, Richard, H. (2004). "Mental Accounting, Saving and Self Control." *Advances in Behavioral Economics*. Colin F. Camerer, George Loewenstein, and Matthew Rabin (eds.). Russell Sage Foundation. Princeton, NJ: Princeton University Press, 395-428.

Shiv, B. & Fedorikhin, A. (1999). "Heart and Mind in Conflict: Interplay of Affect and Cognition in Consumer Decision Making." *Journal of Consumer Research*, *Vol. 26*, 278-282.

Smith, T. G. (2004). "The McDonald's Equilibrium: Advertising, Empty Calories, and the Endogenous Determination of Dietary Preferences." *Social Choice and Welfare*, *Vol. 23*, No. 3, 383-413.

Smith, Trenton. (2002). "The McDonald's Equilibrium: Advertising, Empty Calories, and the Endogenous Determination of Dietary Preferences." Department of Economics, University of California, Santa Barbara.

Smith, Trenton & Tasnadi, A. (2007). "A Theory of Natural Addiction." *Games and Economic Behavior*. Available at SSRN: http://ssrn.com/abstract=979192.

Strahilevitz, M. A. & Myers, J. G. (1998). "Donations to Charity as Purchase Incentives: How Well They Work May Depend on What You Are Trying to Sell." *Journal of Consumer Research*, *Vo. 24*, 434-446.

Strotz, R. H. (1955). "Myopia and Inconsistency in Dynamic Utility Maximization." *The Review of Economic Studies*, *Vol. 23*, 165-180.

Stroebele, N. & de Castro, J. M. (2004). "The Effect of Ambience on Food Intake and Food Choice." *Nutrition*, *Vol. 20*, 821-838.

Terry, K. & Beck, S. (1985). "Eating Style and Food Storage Habits in the Home—Assessment of Obese and Nonobese Families." *Behavior Modification*, *Vol. 9*, 242-261.

Thaler, Richard H. (1980). "Towards a Positive Theory of Consumer Choice." *Journal of Economic Behavior and Organization*, *Vol. 1*, 39-60.

Thaler, Richard, H. (1981). "Some Empirical Evidence on Dynamic Inconsistency." *Economic Letters*, *Vol. 8*, 201-207.

Thaler, Richard H. (2004). "Mental Accounting Matters." *Advances in Behavioral Economics*. Colin F. Camerer, George Loewenstein, and Matthew Rabin (eds.). Russell Sage Foundation. Princeton, NJ: Princeton University Press, 74-103.

Thaler, R. H. & Shefrin, H. M. (1981). "An Economic Theory of Self Control." *Journal of Political Economy*, *Vol. 89*, 392-406.

Thaler, Richard, H. & Shlomo Benartzi. (2004). "Save More Tomorrow (TM): Using Behavioral Economics To Increase Employee Saving." *Journal of Political Economy*, University of Chicago Press, *Vol. 112(S1)*, S164-S187, February.

Tuorila, H. M., et al. (1998). "Effect of Expectations and the Definition of Product Category on the Acceptance of Unfamiliar Foods." *Food Quality and Preference*, *Vol. 9*, 421-430.

U.S. Department of Agriculture, Food and Nutrition Service. (2006)., National School Lunch Program fact sheet. Available at: http://www.fns.usda.gov/cnd/lunch/AboutLunch/NSLPFactSheet.pdf.

Variyam, J. N. (February 2005). "The Price is Right: Economics and the Rise in Obesity." *Amber Waves*, *3(1)*, 20-27.

Variyam, J. N. & Cawley, J. (2006). "*Nutrition Labels and Obesity*." National Bureau of Economic Research Working Paper 11956, National Bureau of Economic Research, Inc., Cambridge, MA.

Volkow, N. D., et al. (2002). "Non-Hedonic' Food Motivation in Humans Involves Dopamine in the Dorsal Striatum and Methylphenidate Amplifies This Effect." *Synapse*, *Vol. 44*, 175-180.

Walker, Rob. (2004). "The Hidden (in Plain Sight) Persuaders." *The New York Times*, December 5.

Wansink, B. (1994). "Antecedents and Mediators of Eating Bouts." *Family and Consumer Sciences Research Journal, Vol. 23*, 166-182.

Wansink, B. (1996). "Can Package Size Accelerate Consumption Volume?" *Journal of Marketing, Vol. 60*, 1-14.

Wansink, B. (2004). "Environmental Factors That Increase the Food Intake and Consumption Volume of Unknowing Consumers," *Annual Review of Nutrition, Vol. 24*, 455-479.

Wansink, B. (2006). *Mindless Eating: Why We Eat More Than We Think*. New York: Bantam Dell.

Wansink, B. & Deshpande, R. (1994). "'Out of Sight Out of Mind': The Impact of Household Stockpiling on Usage Rates." *Marketing Letters, Vol. 5*, 91-100.

Wansink, B. & Kim, J. (2004). "Bad Popcorn in Big Buckets: Portion Size Can Influence Intake As Much As Taste." *Journal of Nutrition Education Behavior*, September-October, *Vol. 37*, No. 5, 242-245.

Wansink, B. & Linder, L. R. (2003). "Interactions Between Forms of Fat Consumption and Restaurant Bread Consumption." *International Journal of Obesity, Vol. 27*, 866-868.

Wansink, B. & van Ittersum, K. (2003). "Bottoms Up! The Influence of Elongation on Pouring and Consumption." *Journal of Consumer Research, Vol. 30*, 455-463.

Welsh, D., Davis, C. & Shaw, A. (1993). *USDA's Food Guide: Background and Development*. Miscellaneous Publication No. 1514. U.S. Department of Agriculture, Human Nutrition Information Service.

Wilde, P. E. & Ranney, C. K. (2000). "The Monthly Food Stamp Cycle: Shopping Frequency and Food Intake Decisions in an Endogenous Switching Regression Gramwork. *American Journal of Agricultural Economics, Vol. 82*, No. 1, 200-213.

Young, L. R. & Nestle, M. (2002). "The Contribution of Expanding Portions Sizes To the U.S. Obesity Epidemic." *American Journal of Public Health, Vol. 92*, 246-249.

End Notes

[1] There are competing explanations for this behavior, flat-rate biases being one of them. Others include the possi-bility that people underestimate the future utility received from a service

and that individuals may choose to overpay upfront as a commitment mechanism to influence future behavior.

[2] Though carbonated soft drinks are not a choice within the actual school meal programs, they are available for purchase at some schools. Some cafe-terias do offer other sugary beverages a la carte.

[3] Evidence that stockpiling food leads to increased consumption in the short run may offer another explanation for the finding by Shapiro (2005)—that consumption patterns among food stamp recipients challenge the assump-tion of exponential discounting.

In: Maintaining a Healthy Diet
Editor: Anna R. Bernstein

ISBN: 978-1-60741-856-6

Chapter 3

DIETARY ASSESSMENT OF MAJOR TRENDS IN U.S. FOOD CONSUMPTION, 1970-2005

United States Department of Agriculture

ABSTRACT

This report examines major trends in the amount of food available for consumption in the United States between 1970 and 2005 using data from the ERS Food Availability (Per Capita) Data System. The report also estimates whether Americans are meeting Federal dietary recommendations for each of the major food groups by comparing the data with dietary recommendations in the *2005 Dietary Guidelines for Americans* and the MyPyramid Food Guidance System. Findings show that Americans do not meet the Federal dietary recommendations. In order to meet them, Americans would need to substantially lower their intake of added fats, refined grains, and added sugars and sweeteners and increase their consumption of fruits, vegetables, whole grains, and low-fat milk and milk products.

Keywords: Agriculture, added fats and oils, added sugars and sweeteners, dairy, *Dietary Guidelines for Americans*, dietary recommendations, eggs, food, food consumption, fruits, meat, MyPyramid Food Guidance System, nutrients, grains, nuts, vegetables.

ACKNOWLEDGMENTS

The authors gratefully acknowledge the valuable assistance and data from Mark Ash, Allen Baker, Don Blayney, Nathan Childs, Erik Dohlman, Steve Haley, David Harvey, Alberto Jerardo, Keithly Jones, Gary Lucier, Agnes Perez, Susan Pollack, Fawzi Taha, and Gary Vocke from the U.S. Department of Agriculture, Economic Research Service, and Steve Koplin from the U.S. Department of Commerce, National Oceanic and Atmospheric Administration.

SUMMARY

The U.S. obesity rate among adults has more than doubled since 1970. The extent of obesity in this country has focused attention on what Americans have been eating. Americans are eating more from all of the major food groups—even fruits and vegetables. However, many are not meeting the Federal dietary recommendations. For Americans to meet these recommendations, they would need to substantially lower their intake of added fats, refined grains, and added sugars and sweeteners and increase their consumption of fruits, vegetables, whole grains, and lower fat milk and milk products.

What Is the Issue?

According to the National Center for Health Statistics, about two-thirds of U.S. adults in 2003-04 were either overweight or obese, compared with 47 percent in 1976-80. During the same period, the obesity rate among adult Americans has more than doubled, from 15 percent to 32 percent. This raises questions about what and how much Americans are consuming each year.

What Did the Study Find?

ERS's food availability data suggest that the food available for consumption increased since 1970 for all major food groups. Although availability continued to rise in the last three decades, many Americans still fall short of Federal dietary recommendations for certain food groups.

According to ERS's loss-adjusted food availability data, Americans are consuming too many foods and beverages high in fats and carbohydrates and too few nutrient-dense foods and beverages, such as lower fat milk and milk prod-ucts, fruits, and vegetables.

Grains

Total grain availability (wheat flour, rice, corn products, oat prod-ucts, and barley products) increased 41 percent, from 137 pounds per person in 1970 to 192 pounds per person in 2005. For Americans on a 2,000-calorie-per-day diet, the *2005 Dietary Guidelines for Americans* recommend consumption of 6 ounce-equivalents (oz-eq) of grains per day with whole grains accounting for at least half of this amount. Using ERS's loss-adjusted food availability data, the researchers estimated that Americans on a 2,000-calorie-per day diet consumed 8.1 oz-eq of grains per person per day in 2005 of which 7.2 oz-eq were refined grains and 0.9 oz-eq were whole grains. This suggests that Americans, on average, over-consume refined grains yet fall short on whole-grain intake.

Fruits and Vegetables

In 2005, the amount of fruits and vegetables avail-able per person for consumption reached 687 pounds (fresh weight equiva-lent), 19 percent above the 1970 level. The *Dietary Guidelines* recommend that Americans eat 2 cups of fruits and 2.5 cups of vegetables per person per day as part of a 2,000-calorie-per-day diet. The loss-adjusted food availability data suggest that Americans on a 2,000-calorie-per-day diet consumed 0.9 cup of fruits and 1.7 cups of vegetables per person per day in 2005. Thus, Americans, on average, are eating less than the recommended amounts.

Milk and Milk Products

The availability of all milk and milk products increased 6 percent, from 564 pounds per person (milk equivalent) in 1970 to about 601 pounds per person in 2005. The 2005 *Dietary Guidelines* recommend that Americans consume 3 cups of milk and milk products per person per day as part of a 2,000-calorie-per-day diet. Using the loss-adjusted food availability data, the researchers estimated that Americans on a 2,000-calorie-per-day diet consumed 1.8 cups of milk and milk products per person per day in 2005, suggesting that Americans, on average, are consuming too little.

Added Fats and Oils

The *Dietary Guidelines* recommend that Americans keep total fat consumption between 20 and 35 percent of daily energy intake. In 2005, total added fats and oils available for consumption reached 86 pounds per person compared with 53 pounds per person in 1970. This 2005 estimate translates into 71.6 grams of added fats and oils per person per day after adjusting for plate waste and other losses. This estimate does not include dietary fats that occur naturally in foods, such as in dairy prod-ucts and meats. Added fats and oils account for about 32 percent of total calories for a 2,000-calorie-per-day diet. In short, the findings suggest that Americans, on average, need to cut back on added fats and oils because, while the 32-percent figure is within the *Guidelines'* range, it includes only added fats and oils and excludes fats and oils naturally present in some foods.

Meat, Eggs, and Nuts

The total amount of meat, eggs, and nuts available for consumption grew from 225 pounds per person in 1970 to about 242 pounds per person in 2005. The *Dietary Guidelines* recommend 5.5 oz-eq from the meat and beans group per person per day as part of a 2,000-calorie-per-day diet. According to the loss-adjusted food availability data, Americans on a 2,000-calorie-per-day diet consumed an estimated 6.5 oz-eq of meat, poultry, fish, eggs, and nuts per person per day in 2005. This suggests that Americans, on average, eat more than the recommended amount from this food group.

Added Sugars and Sweeteners

In 2005, added sugars and sweeteners available for consumption totaled 142 pounds per person, up 19 percent since 1970. The *Dietary Guidelines* do not provide quantitative recommen-dations for added sugars but rather advise Americans to choose and prepare foods and beverages with little added sugars or caloric sweeteners. The *Guidelines* do, however, suggest that Americans on a 2,000-calorie-per-day diet, who divide their discretionary calorie allowance equally between solid fats and added sugars, limit consumption of added sugars and sweeteners to 8 teaspoons per day. According to the loss-adjusted food availability data, Americans consumed 30 teaspoons per person per day of added sugars and sweeteners in 2005. This finding suggests that Americans, on average, need to scale back on added sugars and sweeteners.

How Was the Study Conducted?

The analysis used the three data series that comprise ERS's Food Availability (Per Capita) Data System to analyze the amount of food available for consumption and the dietary status of Americans. The first series, the core Food Availability data, is the only source of time series data on the food available for human consumption in the United States. This series measures supplies moving through production and trade channels for domestic consumption. It is not a direct measure of actual consumption but is useful to understand trends over time. The analysis used this series to examine the amount of food available for consumption per capita.

The second series, the Loss-Adjusted Food Availability data, adjusts the Food Availability data for spoilage and other losses and converts the data to daily per capita amounts for comparison with Federal dietary recommendations. This series is useful in approximating the amount of food Americans, on average, consume on a daily basis and in estimating whether Americans are meeting the Federal dietary recommendations for each food group and for oils.

The third series, the Nutrient Availability data, calculated by USDA's Center for Nutrition Policy and Promotion, uses the Food Availability data to calcu-late the amounts per capita per day of food energy (calories) and 27 nutri-ents and dietary components (i.e., protein, carbohydrates, fats, vitamins, and minerals) in the Nation's food supply. The analysis used the nutrient availability data to estimate the percent of calories contributed by fat and satu-rated fat in the average American's diet.

INTRODUCTION

According to the National Center for Health Statistics, about two-thirds of U.S. adults in 2003-04 were either overweight or obese, compared with 47 percent in 1976-1980. The U.S. obesity rate among adults has more than doubled, from 15 percent in 1976-1980 to 32 percent in 2003-04. The extent of obesity has focused attention on what Americans have been eating. The main reason for this weight gain is the estimated increase in caloric intake without a corresponding increase in physical activity. More than 50 percent of U.S. adults are not physically active. Poor diets and sedentary lifestyles have been associated with diet-related chronic diseases in adults that include hypertension, type 2 diabetes, cardiovascular disease, and certain kinds of cancer (HHS, 2005).

In an effort to promote a healthy, balanced diet with adequate physical activity and to reduce the incidence of diet-related health conditions, the U.S. Department of Agriculture and U.S. Department of Health and Human Services publish jointly the *Dietary Guidelines for Americans*. Since its inception in 1980, the *Guidelines* has been published every 5 years to provide targeted dietary recommendations for Americans over 2 years of age. Although the core dietary messages have remained constant over time (e.g., eat more vegetables), each edition differs slightly to reflect the latest scientific and medical information on nutrition and health. For example, the January 2005 *Guidelines* and a supporting guidance document, the MyPyramid Food Guidance System, introduced specific recommendations for whole-grain consumption. The 2005 edition also breaks down the new daily recommendations into 12 calorie levels ranging from 1,000 to 3,200 calories per day, depending on age, gender, and level of physical activity (table 1). The MyPyramid Food Guidance System replaced the 1992 Food Guide Pyramid and is designed to help Americans consume the recom-mended amounts of the different food groups.

Among the major recommendations in 2005:

- Grains—emphasize that at least half of total grains consumed should be whole grains,
- Vegetables—emphasize dark green vegetables, orange vegetables, and legumes (i.e., dry beans, peas, or lentils[1]),
- Fruits—emphasize variety and "go easy" on fruit juices,
- Milk—emphasize fat-free and low-fat milk and milk products,
- Meat and beans—emphasize low-fat and lean meats, nuts, seeds, and legumes, and
- Oils[2]—use mostly monounsaturated and polyunsaturated fats, such as those found in fish, nuts, and vegetable oils and de-emphasize solid fats, such as butter, margarine, shortening, and lard.

Table 1. Daily amount of Food from Each Group as Recommended by the USDA Food Pyramid Guide in the 2005 Dietary Guidelines for Americans

Food group	1,000	1,200	1,400	1,600	1,800	Calorie level[1] 2,000	2,200	2,400	2,600	2,800	3,000	3,200
	Number											
Fruits[2] (cups)	1	1	1.5	1.5	1.5	2	2	2	2	2.5	2.5	2.5
Vegetables[3] (cups)	1	1.5	1.5	2	2.5	2.5	3	3	3.5	3.5	4	4
Grains[4]	3	4	5	5	6	6	7	8	9	10	10	10
[Whole-grain portion (oz-eq)]	1.5	2	2.5	3	3	3	3.5	4	4.5	5	5	5
Meat and beans[5] (oz-eq)	2	3	4	5	5	5.5	6	6.5	6.5	7	7	7
Milk[6] (cups)	2	2	2	3	3	3	3	3	3	3	3	3
Oils[7] (tsp)	3	4	4	5	5	6	6	7	8	8	10	11
Discretionary calorie allowance[8]	165	171	171	132	195	267	290	362	410	426	512	648

Note: oz-eq = ounce-equivalent.

[1] Calorie levels are set across a wide range to accommodate the needs of different individuals. This table can be used to help assign individualsto the food intake pattern at a particular calorie level. A 2,000-calorie-per-day level is used in this report to be consistent with the nutrition factslabels found on packaged foods.

[2] The fruit group includes all fresh, frozen, canned, and dried fruits and fruit juices. In general, 1 cup of fruit or 100 percent fruit juice, or 1/2 cupof dried fruit can be considered as 1 cup from the fruit group.

[3] The vegetable group includes all fresh, frozen, canned, and dried vegetables and vegetable juices. In general, 1 cup of raw or cooked vegetables or vegetable juice, or 2 cups of raw leafy greens can be considered as 1 cup from the vegetable group. According to the

MyPyramidPlan, 1 cup of whole, mashed, or cooked dry legumes or 1 cup of 1/2 inch cubes of tofu count as 1 cup from the vegetable group.

[4] The grains group includes all foods made from wheat, rice, oats, cornmeal, and barley—such as bread, pasta, oatmeal, breakfast cereals, tortillas, and grits. In general, 1 slice of bread, 1 cup of ready-to-eat cereal flakes, or 1/2 cup of cooked rice, pasta, or cooked cereal can beconsidered as 1 oz-eq from the grains group. At least half of all grains consumed should be whole grains.

[5] The meat and beans group includes, in general, 1 ounce of lean meat, poultry, or fish, 1 egg, 1 tablespoon peanut butter, 1/4 cup cooked dry beans, or 1/2 ounce of nuts or seeds.

[6] The milk group includes all fluid milk products and foods made from milk that retain their calcium content, such as yogurt and cheese.Foods made from milk that have little to no calcium, such as cream cheese, cream, and butter, are not part of the group. Most milk group choices should be fat-free or low-fat. In general, 1 cup of milk or yogurt, 1½ ounces of natural cheese, or 2 ounces of processed cheese can be considered as 1 cup from the milk group.

[7] Oils include fats from many different plants and from fish that are liquid at room temperature, such as canola, corn, olive, soybean, and sunflower oil. Some foods are naturally high in oils, like nuts, olives, some fish, and avocados. Foods that are mainly oil include mayonnaise,certain salad dressings, and soft margarine.

[8] Discretionary calorie allowance is the remaining amount of calories in a food intake pattern after accounting for the calories needed for all foodgroups using forms of foods that are fat-free or low-fat and with no added sugars.Source: Prepared by USDA, Economic Reseearch Service using data from Dietary Guidelines for Americans, 2005, Appendix A2 “USDA Food Guide.”

This report updates the analysis of Putnam et al. (2002), which examined overall food consumption patterns between 1970 and 2000. Using the 2000 edition of *Nutrition and Your Health: Dietary Guidelines for Americans*, Putnam et al. estimated whether Americans were meeting the *Guidelines'* recommendations. In this report, we used the 2005 *Dietary Guidelines for Americans* to estimate the dietary status of Americans. The main goals of this study were to: (1) analyze the amount of food available for consump-tion since 1970 for each food group, and (2) estimate whether Americans are meeting the *Guidelines'* recommendations for each food group.

Food consumption patterns change in response to changes in relative food prices, increases in real (adjusted for inflation) disposable income, and food assistance for the poor. Moreover, time series data on actual consumption by Americans are lacking. Most consumer surveys of dietary intake cover 1 or a few years of consumption and most are not nationally representative of the U.S. population. We tracked the amount of food available for consumption over time and the dietary status of Americans using the ERS Food Availability (Per Capita) Data System, a unique, popular, and often-cited data system that provides proxies for actual consumption.[3] The data system contains three separate but related data series—the Food Availability data, the Loss-Adjusted Food Availability data, and the Nutrient Availability data—that each look at food consumption differently.

The first series, the core food availability data, is the only time series data on the amount of food available for consumption in the United States and is a continuous series extending back to 1909 for many commodities. The data are calculated for each food or commodity (e.g., beef, low-fat milk, and fresh broccoli) as the sum of annual production, beginning stocks, and imports minus exports, ending stocks, and nonfood uses. Per capita esti-mates are calculated by dividing the total annual food supply of a commodity by the U.S. population that year. Food availability data do not directly measure actual consumption but rather serve as useful indicators of food consumption trends over time. Used in this manner, the data provide an upper bound on the amount of food available for consumption.

The second series, the loss-adjusted food availability data, adjusts the food availability data for spoilage and other losses and converts the per capita data to MyPyramid equivalents or daily allowance for comparison with Federal dietary recommendations. The percentage of food lost due to spoilage and other losses at several different stages along the food produc-tion, marketing, and consumption chain are identified for each commodity or food. In addition, the estimates incorporate loss assumptions for non-edible food parts, such as rinds, seeds, cores, and stems, as estimated in USDA's *Nutrient Database for Standard Reference* (www.nal. usda.gov/fnic/foodcomp/search). Next, we converted the loss-adjusted data from pounds per capita per year into daily per capita food intake in MyPyramid equivalents or daily allowance (as identified in USDA's *MyPyramid Food Guidance System*, www.Mypyramid.gov). The estimated MyPyramid equivalents for individual commodities or foods are then aggre-gated to determine total daily amounts for each food group. We then compared these estimates with Federal dietary recommendations to provide an estimate of whether Americans are meeting the dietary recommendations for the different food groups.

In particular, we compared the amount of food consumed by the average American with the amount recommended in USDA's Food Guide in Appendix A-2 of the 2005 *Dietary Guidelines for Americans*. These recom-mendations are broken into 12 calorie levels ranging from 1,000 to 3,200 calories per day. Our data are unavailable on the distribution of Americans among each of the 12 calorie levels in the *Dietary Guidelines* so instead, we used the 2,000-calorie-per-day reference level in our analysis to be consis-tent with the level used throughout the examples in the *Dietary Guidelines* and on the nutrition facts labels found on most packaged foods. Like the food availability data series, the loss-adjusted data do not directly measure actual consumption. The data are useful in approximating the amount of food Americans, on average, consume on a daily basis.

The third series, the nutrient availability data, calculated by USDA's Center for Nutrition Policy and Promotion (www.cnpp.usda.gov), uses the food availability data to calculate the amounts per capita per day of food energy (calories) and 27 nutrients and dietary components (i.e., protein, carbohy-drates, fats, vitamins, and minerals) in the Nation's food supply. As with the food availability data, the resulting nutrient and calorie estimates do not account for losses due to the household and marketing system. In our analysis, we used the nutrient availability data to estimate the percentage of calories contributed by fat and saturated fat in the average American's diet.

The analyses had several key findings. We found that many Americans do not meet the Federal daily dietary recommendations.They consume foods and beverages high in fats and carbohydrates at greater than recommended rates and nutrient-dense foods and beverages, such as lower fat milk and milk products, fruits, and vegetables at levels below recommended rates (fig. 1).

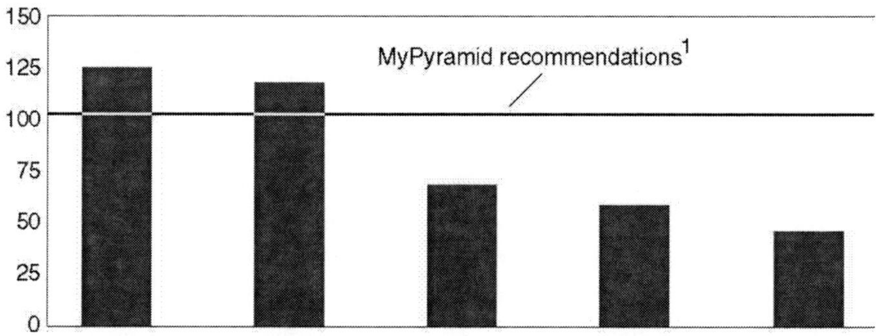

[1]2005 data based on a 2,000-calorie diet.
Source: USDA, ERS Food Availability (Per Capita) Data System.

Figure 1. Loss-adjusted per capita food availabiity out of balance with dietary recommendations Percent of recommendation

Not Enough Whole Grains

The total amount of food grains available for consumption in the United States increased 41 percent over the past three decades according to ERS's food availability data. Grain availability grew from 137 pounds per person (unadjusted for waste and spoilage) in 1970 to 192 pounds in 2005 (table 2). Of this 56-pound increase, 36 percent was from corn products (snacks, for example), 34 percent was from white and whole-wheat flour, 24 percent was from rice, and 8 percent was from durum flour (pasta, for example). Estimated availability of rye flour, barley products, and oat products remained relatively constant. Although the amount of rice and corn products available for consumption almost tripled between 1970 and 2005, the relative importance of the different food grains remained unchanged, with wheat maintaining its dominant share of total grains available for consumption (fig. 2).

The 2005 *Dietary Guidelines* provided, for the first time, specific dietary recommendations for whole grains. The *Guidelines* recommend that half of the daily grain allowance be from whole grains. For example, the *Guidelines* recommend that Americans on a 2,000-calorie-per-day diet consume 6 ounce-equivalents (oz-eq) of grains per day, at least 3 oz-eq of which should be whole grains. The goal of the recommendation is to encourage Americans to eat more whole grains for their nutritional benefits. Whole grains are good sources of fiber and other nutrients, such as calcium, magnesium, and potassium. Daily intake of at least 3 oz-eq or more of whole grains per day may help an individual with weight control and can reduce the risk of several chronic diseases.

According to ERS's loss-adjusted food availability data, Americans, on average, consumed 7.5 oz-eq of grains per day, mostly refined grains. The database has some significant data gaps for whole grains, such as popcorn, wheat products, and other products, and, therefore, the data do not provide a comprehensive estimate of the per capita consumption of whole grains. When considering both the whole grains covered in the data and those omitted, we estimate that Americans consume 0.9 oz-eq of whole grains—a far cry from the recommended 3 oz-eq of whole-grains for a 2,000-calorie-per-day diet.[4] Also, if we add the estimated 0.6 oz-eq from the missing whole-grain foods to the 7.5 oz-eq included in the database, we estimate that the new total for grains would be 8.1 oz-eq in 2005. In short, we found that Americans are eating more than double the recommended amount of refined grains per day while eating a third of the recommended amount of whole grains.

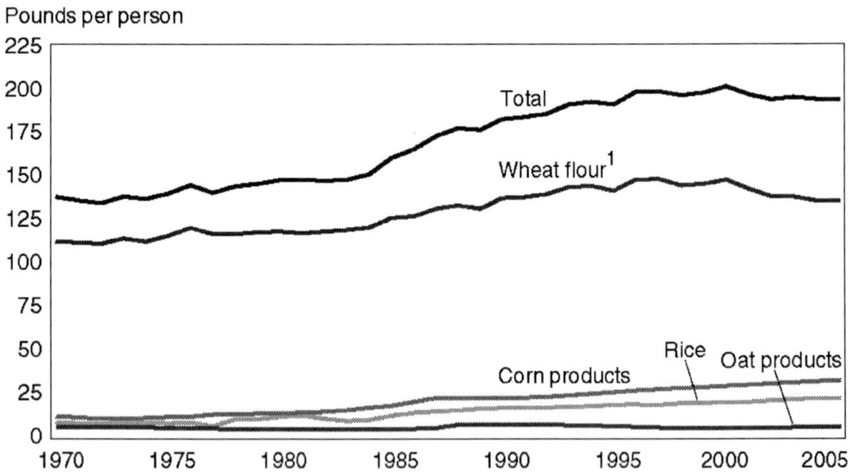

[1]2005 data based on a 2,000-calorie diet.

Source: USDA, ERS Food Availability (Per Capita) Data System.

Figure 2. Per capita total grain availability grew by 55 pounds between 1970 and 2005

Table 2. Per Capita Availability of Grains Grew 41 Percent between 1970 and 2005

Item	Per capita availability[1]		Change, 1970 to 2005	2005 loss-adjusted food availability[2]
	1970	2005		
	Pounds		Percent	Oz-eq/day
Total wheat flour	110.9	134.1	21	5.1
White and whole wheat flour	104.0	122.3	18	4.8
Durum wheat flour[3]	6.9	11.8	71	.4
Rye flour	1.2	.5	-58	---
Rice (milled)	6.8	21.0	177	.6
Total corn products	11.1	31.4	183	1.6
Corn flour and meal	7.0	18.8	169	.9
Hominy and grits	2.2	8.1	268	.4
Corn starch	1.9	4.5	137	.3
Oat products	4.7	4.6	-3	.1
Barley products	1.0	.7	-34	---
Total flour and cereal products[4]	136.5	192.3	41	8.1

Notes: Totals may not add due to rounding. Oz-eq = ounce equivalent. = less than 0.05 oz-eq.

[1] Aggregate data, unadjusted for cooking losses, plate waste, and other losses, excluding quantities used in alcoholic beverages and fuel, popcorn, and other whole-grain foods.

[2] Adjusted for cooking losses, plate waste, and other losses. According to MyPyramid Plan, 1 slice of bread, 1 cup of ready-to-eat cereal flakes, or 1/2 cup of cooked rice, pasta, or cookedcereal can be considered as 1 oz-eq from the grains group. At least half of all grains consumed should be whole grains.

[3] Includes flour equivalent of imported pasta products.

[4] The estimate of 8.1 oz-eq is the 7.5 oz-eq from the loss-adjusted food availability data plus themissing whole-grain foods of 0.6 oz-eq from Putnam et al. (2002).Source: USDA, ERS Food Availability (Per Capita) Data System.

AMERICANS ARE CONSUMING MORE FRUITS AND VEGETABLES

In general, Americans have been consuming more fruits and vegetables over the last three decades, according to food availability data. In 2005, per capita total fruit and vegetable availability (fresh and processed, fresh weight equivalent, unadjusted for waste and spoilage) reached 687 pounds, up 110 pounds, or 19 percent, since 1970. This 19-percent increase was not distributed equally among the 134 fruits and vegetables covered in the ERS data. Much of the rise within fruits was contributed by the noncitrus group, particularly apples, bananas, and grapes (table 3). Among the vegetable group, tomatoes, onions, and leafy lettuces contributed to the increase (table 4).

Despite our estimate that Americans are consuming more fruits and vegeta-bles than they did in 1970, they are still not meeting the *Dietary Guidelines'* recommendations. According to the loss-adjusted food availability data, Americans on a 2,000-calorie-per-day diet consumed 0.9 cup of fresh and processed fruits per person per day in 2005, less than half the *Guidelines'* recommendation of 2 cups. We also estimated that each American ate 1.7 cups of fresh and processed vegetables per day in 2005, about 45 percent below the recommended amount of 2.5 cups in the *Dietary Guidelines*.

The Guidelines also recommend choosing a variety of types of fruits andvegetables because some fruits and vegetables are higher in certain vitaminsand minerals than others. In particular, the Guidelinesencourage Americansto select from all five vegetable subgroups several times a week becauseeach subgroup provides a somewhat different array of nutrients. Forexample, the recommended weekly intake of vegetables for persons on a2,000-calorie-per-day diet consists of dark-green vegetables (3 cups), orangevegetables (2 cups), legumes (i.e., dry beans, peas, and lentils) (3 cups),starchy vegetables (3 cups), and other vegetables (6.5 cups). Of the fivevegetable subgroups, starchy vegetables, particularly potatoes, dominatedvegetable consumption, accounting for approximately a third of the total andslightly above the recommended level (fig. 3). Legumes had the lowest esti-mated consumption level. Overall, Americans consumed a limited variety of vegetables.

Table 3. Per Capita Availability of Fruits Increased 13 Percent between 1970 and 2005

	Per capita availability[1]		Change, 1970 to 2005	2005 loss-adjusted food availability[2]
	1970	2005		
	Pounds,	*fresh-weight equivalent*	*Percent*	*Cups/day*
Citrus, melons, and berries[3,4]	138.8	136.4	-2	0.36
Citrus	113.7	101.2	-11	.26
Fresh	28.8	21.6	-25	.06
Processed (juice)	84.9	79.6	-6	.20
Melons[3]	21.6	25.8	19	.05
Watermelon	13.5	13.8	2	.03
Cantaloup	7.2	10.1	40	.02
Berries[3]	3.5	8.9	156	.05
Fresh and frozen strawberries	2.9	7.7	163	.03
Other fruits[3,4]	101.9	136.0	36	.57
Fresh bananas	17.4	25.1	45	.08
Fresh apples	17.2	16.9	-1	.12
Fresh grapes	2.9	8.6	197	.04
Apple juice	6.4	22.5	254	.07
Grape juice	2.4	5.6	135	.02
Canned applesauce	5.7	4.3	-24	.07
Canned olives	1.0	1.4	48	.03
Canned peaches	6.8	3.3	-50	.01
Raisins	5.8	7.3	25	.02
Total fruits	240.7	272.4	13	.92

Note: Totals may not add due to rounding.

[1] Aggregate data, unadjusted for cooking losses, plate waste, and other losses.

[2] Adjusted for cooking losses, plate waste, and other losses. According to MyPyramid Plan, 1 cup of fruit or 100% fruit juice, or 1/2 cup of dried fruit can be considered as 1 cup from thefruit group.

[3] Includes food item(s) not shown separately.

[4] Includes fresh and processed fruits.

Source: USDA, ERS Food Availability (Per Capita) Data System.

Table 4. Per Capita Availability of Vegetables Increased 23 Percent between 1970 and 2005

Item	Per capita availability[1]		Change, 1970 to 2005	2005 loss-adjusted food availability[2]
	1970	2005		
	Pounds	*fresh-weight equivalent*	*Percent*	*Cups/day*
Dark-green vegetables[3,4]	3.8	20.2	425	0.16
Leafy lettuces[5]	.6	10.9	1,856	.08
Broccoli	1.5	8.3	446	.04
Deep-yellow vegetables[3,4]	15.0	21.4	43	.10
Carrots	9.5	11.9	24	.06
Sweet potatoes	5.4	4.5	-17	.02
Other starchy vegetables[3,4]	155.5	155.5		.63
Potatoes	121.7	125.6	3	.55
Corn	27.8	26.9	-3	.06
Other vegetables[3,4]	154.9	210.5	36	.80
Head lettuce	22.4	21.1	-6	.12
Canned tomatoes	62.1	73.6	18	.13
Garlic	.4	2.4	450	.01
Fresh tomatoes	12.1	20.2	66	.07
Fresh onions	10.1	21.0	107	.07
Cucumbers	8.5	10.2	20	.03
Bell peppers	2.2	7.1	227	.03
Cabbage	11.0	9.3	-15	.06
Celery	7.3	5.9	-19	.04
Total vegetables	336.8	414.6	23	1.72

Notes: Totals may not add due to rounding. --- = less than 0.5 percent.

[1] Aggregate data, unadjusted for cooking losses, plate waste, and other losses.

[2] Adjusted for cooking losses, plate waste, and other losses. According to MyPyramid Plan, 1 cup of raw or cooked vegetables or vegetable juice, or 2 cups of raw leafy greens can be considered as 1 cup from the vegetable group.

[3] Includes food item(s) not shown separately.

[4] Includes fresh and processed vegetables.

[5] Includes escarole and romaine.

Source: USDA, ERS Food Availability (Per Capita) Data System.

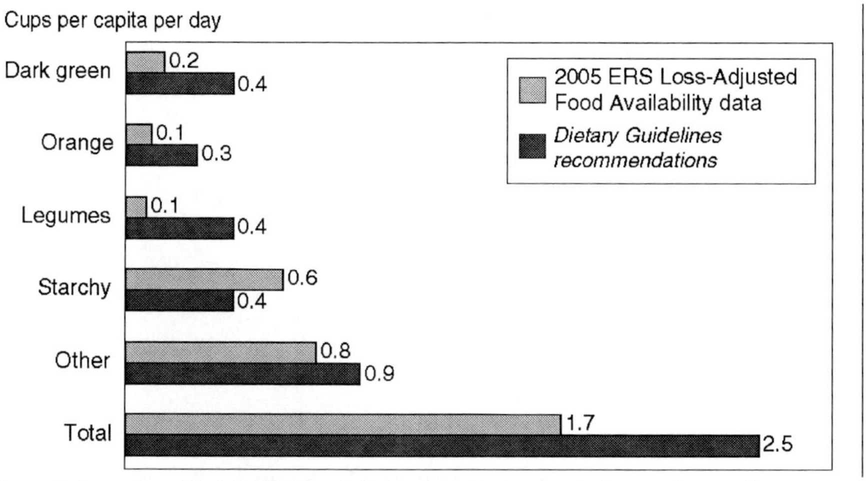

Note: Other vegetables include artichokes, asparagus, snap beans, broccoli, tomatoes, etc.

Source: USDA, ERS Food Availability (Per Capita) DataSystem.

Figure 3. 2005 loss-adjusted food availability data compared with 2005 *Dietary Guidelines'* recommendations for a 2,000-calorie diet

Like vegetable consumption, the bulk of fruit consumption came from a limited variety of fresh and processed fruits. For example, 5 out of the 62 items covered in the loss-adjusted food availability data accounted for more than half (54 percent) of daily fruit intake in 2005—orange juice (20 percent), fresh apples (13 percent), bananas (9 percent), apple juice (8 percent), and fresh grapes (5 percent).

Americans Are Consuming Less Milk but More Cheese

According to the food availability data, the availability of all milk and milk products increased 6 percent between 1970 and 2005, from 564 pounds per person (milk equivalent) to about 601 pounds (table 5). Cheese availability contributed significantly to the increase. Part of this increase can be attrib-uted to the growth of food consumed away from home and the introduction of new, convenient cheese products, such as resealable bags of shredded cheese (Buzby, 2005). Between 1970 and 2005, the availability of cheese (other than cottage cheese) nearly tripled, from 11 pounds per person to 31 pounds per person. Yogurt availability grew about tenfold. Meanwhile, avail-ability of beverage milk, frozen dairy products, dry milk, and evaporated/condensed milk declined. Beverage milk availability decreased 33 percent between 1970 and 2005. Within the beverage milk category, whole-milk availability dropped 73 percent while lower fat milk rose 143 percent (fig. 4). Similarly, availability of frozen dairy products decreased 6 percent, dry milk 45 percent, and evaporated/condensed milk 52 percent.

The 2005 *Dietary Guidelines* recommend that Americans on a 2,000-calorie-per-day diet consume 3 cups of milk and milk products per day. According to our loss-adjusted food availability data, Americans consumed 1.8 cups of milk and milk products per person per day in 2005.[5]

The *Guidelines* also recommend fat-free or low-fat milk or equivalent milk products instead of dairy products high in saturated fat. Food availability data measure reduced-fat and non-fat versions for some dairy products, such as fluid milk, cottage cheese, dry milk, and condensed/evaporated milks, which contributed about a third of the total dairy allowance per person per day. The data do not, however, distinguish the fat content of other dairy products, particularly how much of the increase in cheese consumption is due to the increased use of reduced-fat, low-fat, and non-fat cheese. According to the International Dairy Foods Association, reduced-fat, low-fat, and non-fat cheeses' share of supermarket sales of cheese increased from 19 percent in 1999 to 25 percent in 2005, suggesting that 75 percent of cheese consumption still comes from regular or full-fat cheese products. While Americans are gradually increasing their intake of lower fat cheeses, they need to cut back considerably on higher or full-fat versions of dairy products in order to meet the dietary recommendations.

ADDED FATS AND OILS ALONE CONTRIBUTED 32 PERCENT OF TOTAL CALORIES

Added fats and oils are found in processed food products (e.g., french fries, baked goods, and snacks) and are used for cooking. These fats and oils are consumed in addition to fats that occur naturally in foods, such as in red meat and dairy products. According to the food availability data, per capita availability of added fats and oils (unadjusted for waste and spoilage) reached about 86 pounds per person in 2005, up 33 pounds from 1970. Of the 2005 total, nearly 86 percent consisted of vegetable oils and related products, such as margarine, shortening, and cooking and salad oils. Animal fats, such as butter, lard, and edible tallow, made up the remaining 14 percent (table 6).

One important caveat about the added fats and oils data is that the number of firms reporting vegetable oil production to the U.S. Census Bureau increased noticeably in 2000. As a result, the availability of salad and cooking oils and shortening rose from 50 pounds per person in 1999 to 65 pounds person in 2000, a 31-percent increase. We believe it unlikely that this unusually large increase in the number of firms occurred in 1 year; it is more likely that the number increased incrementally over time. The jump could suggest that the availability estimates in a few years before 2000 were somewhat underestimated. However, we do not have additional information from the U.S. Census Bureau to clarify that supposition. Therefore, the data must be interpreted with care when discussing particular estimates for salad and cooking oils and shortening around 2000 or when discussing more aggregated numbers that use these estimates, such as estimates for total vegetable fats and oils or total added fats and oils seen in figure 5.

In general, the added fats and oils data show modest increases from 1970 to 1999, the big increase in 2000, moderate increases until 2002, and then a decline between 2002 and 2005. Despite the data limitations around 2000, the data make the important point that the availability of added fats and oil has generally trended upward since 1970.

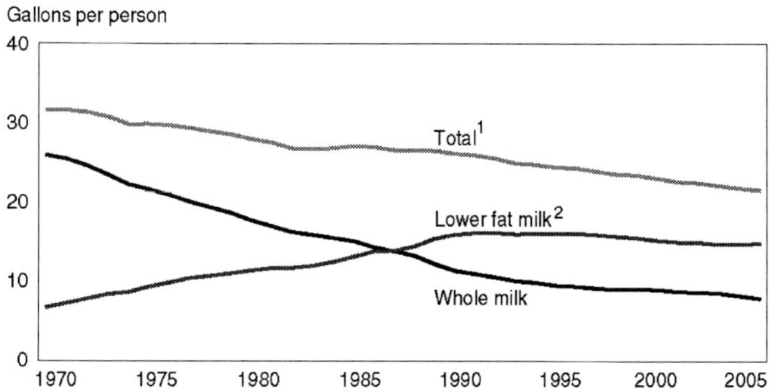

[1] Includes flavored milk and buttermilk.

[2] Includesbuttermilk (1.5 percent fat), plain and flavored reduced-fat milk (2 percent fat), low-fat milk (1 percent fat), and fat-free milk.

Source: USDA, ERS Food Availability (Per Capita) DataSystem.

Figure 4. Per capita availability of whole milk declined 73 percent, while that of lower fat milk grew 143 percent between 1970 and 2005.

Table 5. Per Capita Availability of Milk and Milk Products Increased 6 Percent between 1970 and 2005

Item	Per capita availability[1]		Change, 1970 to 2005	2005 loss-adjusted food availability[2]
	1970	2005		
	Gallons		*Percent*	*Cups/day*
Fluid milk products	31.4	22.3	-30	0.69
Beverage milk	31.3	21.0	-33	.65
Whole	25.5	6.9	-73	.22
Plain	24.8	6.6	-73	.21
Flavored	.7	.3	-55	.01
Lower fat and skim milk	5.8	14.0	143	.43
Plain (2% fat)	3.2	6.9	111	.21
Plain (1% fat)	.2	2.5	1,081	.08
Flavored (1% and 2% fat)	.3	1.4	300	.04
Skim	1.3	3.1	132	.10
Buttermilk	.6	.2	-69	.01
Yogurt	.1	1.0	941	.03
	Pounds		*Percent*	*Cups/day*
Total cheese				
(excl. cream cheese)[3]	16.5	34.0	106	.69
Cheese other than cottage[3,4]	11.4	31.4	176	.68
Cheddar				
Mozzarella				
Cottage cheese	5.8	10.1	75	.24
Frozen dairy products[5] Ice	1.2	10.2	754	.24
cream	5.2	2.6	-50	.01
Low-fat ice cream Frozen	28.5	24.1	-15	.10
yogurt and other misc.	17.8	15.4	-13	.06
Condensed/evaporated	7.7	5.9	-23	.02
milks				
Dry milk	3.0	2.8	-6	.01
	12.0	5.8	-52	.04
	5.8	3.2	-45	.13
Total milk and milk products	563.9	600.5	6	1.77

Note: Totals may not add due to rounding.

[1] Aggregate data, unadjusted for cooking losses, plate waste, and other losses.

[2] Adjusted for cooking losses, plate waste, and other losses. According to MyPyramid Plan, 1 cup of milk or yogurt, 1½ ounces of hard cheese,2 ounces of processed cheese, 2 cups of cottage cheese, or 1½ cups of ice cream can be considered as 1 cup from the milk group. Only themilk portion of half and half and eggnog are included in the daily dairy allowance; the cream portion is included in added fats.

[3] Cream cheese is counted in added fats. 4Excludes full-skim American, cottage, pot, and baker's cheese. 5Includes items not shown separately, such as mellorine, which is a nondairy alternative to ice cream (1970-1990).

Source: USDA, ERS Food Availability (Per Capita) Data System.

Table 6. Per Capita Availability of Added Fats and Oils up 63 Percent between 1970 and 2005

Item	Per capita availability[1]		Change, 1970 to 2005	2005 loss-adjusted food availability[2]
	1970	2005		
	Pounds	*fat content basis*	*Percent*	*Grams*
Animal fat	14.1	11.8	-17	9.2
Butter	4.3	3.7	-15	3.6
Lard (direct use)[3]	4.6	1.5	-66	1.0
Edible beef tallow (direct use)[3]	NA	3.8	NA	2.3
Shortening[4]	4.7	2.7	-42	2.3
Margarine[4]	.5		-91	
Vegetable fats and oils	38.5	73.7	91	59.6
Salad and cooking oils	15.4	42.7	177	33.5
Shortening	12.6	26.4	109	22.0
Margarine	8.2	3.2	-61	2.3
Other edible fats and oils[5,6]	2.3	1.5	-36	1.7
Dairy fat[7]	--	--	--	2.7
Total added fats and oils[8]	52.6	85.5	63	71.6

Notes: NA = not applicable or not available. --- = less than 0.05. Totals may not add due to rounding.

1 Aggregate data, unadjusted for cooking losses, plate waste, and other losses. Total fats andoils reported on a fat content basis.

2 Adjusted for cooking losses, plate waste, and other losses. Fat content of butter and margarinecalculated at 80 percent. One gram of fat equals 9 calories.

3 Excludes use in margarine and shortening.

4 Animal fat portion for shortening and margarine are 9.4 and 1.3 percent, respectively.

5 In 2000, the number of firms reporting vegetable oil production increased.

6 Specialty fats used mainly in confections and nondairy creamers.

7 Includes only the cream portion of half and half, heavy and light cream, sour cream, and cream cheese.

8 Excludes most naturally occurring fat, such as meats, beverage milks, nuts, and avocados.Source: USDA, ERS Food Availability (Per Capita) Data System.

According to the *Guidelines*, fats are part of a healthful diet, although excessive intake, particularly of saturated fats, is associated with high cholesterol and coronary heart disease. The *Guidelines* recommend that fats and oils, both added and naturally occurring, contribute 20 to 35 percent of daily energy intake depending on calorie level.[6] People on a 2,000-calorieper-day diet, therefore, should consume 400 to 700 calories from fats per day, or 44 to 78 grams of fat. Using the loss-adjusted food availability data, we estimated that Americans consumed 71.6 grams of added fats and oils per person per day in 2005.[7] As previously mentioned, this estimate does not include fats occurring naturally in foods (e.g., in meat and dairy products), yet accounts for about 32 percent of total calories for a 2,000-calorie-per-day diet.

In addition to recommendations for total fat intake, the *Guidelines* suggest limiting saturated fats, found in animal fats, to less than 10 percent of total dietary fat. The *Guidelines* recommend that most fats should be monounsaturated and polyunsaturated fats, such as those found in fish, nuts, and vegetables. According to the nutrient availability data (unadjusted for waste and spoilage), Americans consumed both added and dietary fats in excess of the recommended level. In 2004, per capita total fat (both added and naturally occurring) availability reached 179 grams per day. Of this amount, saturated fats accounted for 31 percent, and unsaturated fats accounted for 69 percent. Therefore, not only do Americans need to decrease their total intake of fat, they also need to substantially lower their intake of saturated fat in order to adhere to the 2005 *Guidelines*.

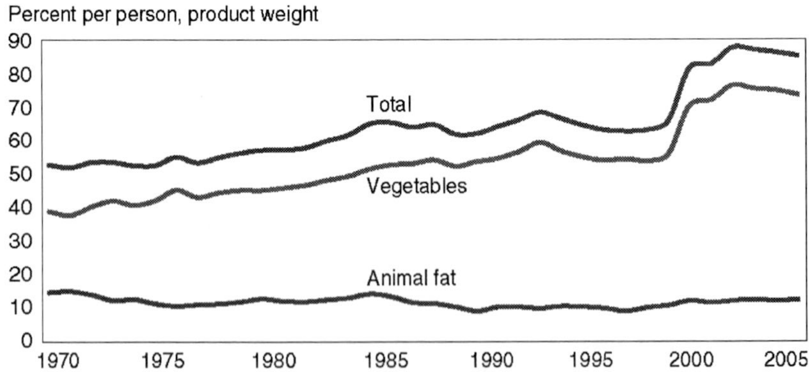

Note: In 2000, there was a dramatic increase in the number of firms reporting vegetable oil production to the U.S. Census Bureau.

Source: USDA, ERS Food Availability (Per Capita) Data System.

Figure 5. Added fats and oils consumption increased 63 percent beween 1970 and 2005

Beef Still Dominates, but Chicken Is Gaining Ground

The total amount of meat, eggs, and nuts available for consumption (unadjusted for waste and spoilage) grew from 225 pounds per person in 1970 to about 242 pounds per person in 2005 according to the food availability data (table 7). This 8-percent increase, however, was not distributed equally across the meat group. Poultry availability, for example, provided a significant contribution to the increase. Between 1970 and 2005, per capita poultry availability more than doubled, from 34 pounds per person to 74 pounds per person. Part of the rise in poultry, particularly chicken, results from the chicken industry's catering to consumers' and foodservice operators' demand for value-added, brand-name, and convenience products (Buzby et al., 2006). During the same period, availability of fish and shellfish and tree nuts and peanuts grew 5 and 3 pounds per person, respectively.

In contrast, red meat availability (beef, veal, pork, and lamb) faced a major decline. Since its peak of 133 pounds per person in 1976, red meat availability fell to 110 pounds per person in 2005. This decline in red meat availability was largely due to beef, which dropped 17 pounds, or 22 percent between 1970 and 2005. Availability of eggs likewise decreased during the same period. Over the past three decades, red meat's share of total meat dropped while the share of poultry continued to rise. However, red meat, particularly beef, remains the main source of protein in Americans' diet (fig. 6).

Ounce for ounce, poultry and fish products have less fat, saturated fat, and cholesterol than beef, according to USDA's Nutrient Database for Standard Reference. Also, according to the nutrient availability data (unadjusted for spoilage and other losses), the proportion of fat in the U.S. food supply contributed by red meat, poultry, and fish declined from 32 percent in 1970 to 20 percent in 2004. Much of this decline can be attributed to red meat's share of fat in the food supply, which dropped from 27 percent to 13 percent during the same period. Similarly, red meat's proportion of saturated fat declined from 35 to 23 percent.

The *Dietary Guidelines* as depicted in the MyPyramid Plan recommends daily consumption of 5.5 oz-eq from the meat and beans group (meat, poultry, fish, legumes, eggs, nuts, and seeds)[8] per person as part of a 2,000calorie-per-day diet. According to the loss-adjusted food availability data, Americans consumed 6.5 oz-eq of meat, poultry, fish, eggs, and nuts per person per day in

2005 (i.e., not including legumes). This estimate is 16 percent above the recommended amount, suggesting that Americans need to decrease their meat intake to meet the recommendations in the *Dietary Guidelines*. In addition, many Americans need to change the types of meats consumed in order to choose diets with less fat, saturated fat, and cholesterol (HHS, 2005).

Table 7. Per Capita Availability of Meat, Eggs, and Nuts[1] Increased 8 Percent between 1970 and 2005

Item	Per capita availability[2]		Change, 1970 to 2005	2005 loss-adjusted food availability[3]
	1970	2005		
	Pounds	*edible weight*	*Percent*	*Oz-eq/day*
Total meat, poultry, and fish[4]	177.5	199.7	13	5.2
Red meat	131.9	110.0	-17	2.9
Beef	79.6	62.4	-22	1.7
Pork	48.1	46.5	-3	1.2
Veal, lamb, and mutton	2.0	.4	-81	
Poultry	33.8	73.6	118	1.8
Chicken	27.4	60.4	120	1.5
Turkey	6.4	13.1	106	.4
Fish and shellfish	11.7	16.1	37	.5
Eggs	39.5	32.7	-17	.5
Nuts (including peanut butter)	7.80	9.87	27	.7
Total meat, eggs, and nuts	224.8	242.3	8	6.5

Notes: Totals may not add due to rounding. Oz-eq = ounce equivalent. --- = less than 0.05.

[1] Legumesare counted in the vegetable group.

[2] Aggregate data, unadjusted for cooking losses, plate waste, and other losses.

[3] Adjusted for cooking losses, plate waste, and other losses. According to MyPyramid, 1 ounceof meat, poultry or fish, ¼ cup cooked dry beans, 1 egg, 1 tablespoon of peanut butter, or ½ounce of nuts or seeds can be considered as 1 oz-eq.

[4] Boneless, trimmed-weight equivalent for the meat group. Excludesall legumes consumed.Legumesare included under the vegetable group in thisanalysis. Total meat group is inpounds.

Source: USDA, ERS Food Availability (Per Capita) DataSystem.

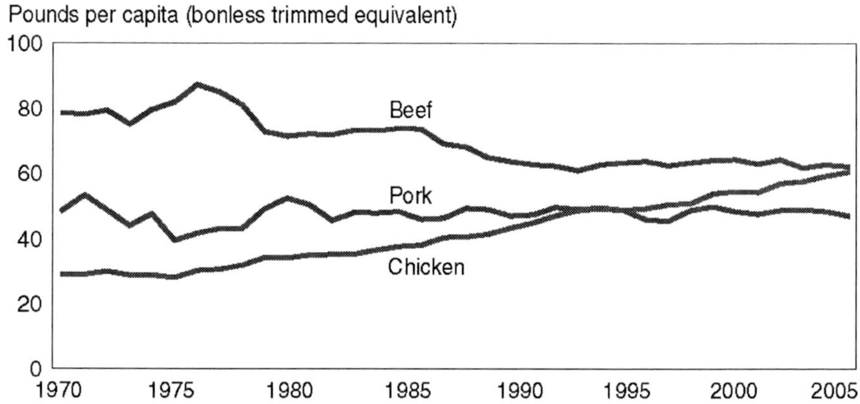

Source: USDA, ERS Food Availability (Per Capita) Data System.

Figure 6. Chicken consumption increased 116 percent between 1970 and 2005.

Added Sugars and Sweeteners Up 19 Percent

Added sugars and sweeteners (or caloric sweeteners) include refined cane and beet sugars, corn sweeteners, and edible syrups added to processed foods and beverages but do not include dietary sugars found naturally in foods, such as in fruits. According to the food availability data, per capita availability of added sugars and sweeteners totaled 142 pounds in 2005, 7 percent less than the 1999 record high of 151 pounds per person, but 19 percent more than in 1970 (table 8).

Perhaps the most interesting change in added sugars and sweeteners between 1970 and 2005 is that annual per capita corn sweetener availability increased 387 percent while per capita availability of refined cane and beet sugars (i.e., sucrose) declined 38 percent (fig. 7). This increase in corn sweeteners was driven mostly by increased use of high-fructose corn syrup (HFCS). Between 1970 and 2005, HFCS's share of all corn sweeteners grew from 3 to 76 percent. Prior to the early 1980s, most food industries used sucrose instead of corn sweeteners. By the mid-1980s, industries had switched to corn sweeteners, particularly HFCS, a low-cost substitute for sugar in beverages. Today, the U.S. soft drink industry is the largest user of HFCS, followed by the processed food and baking industries.

The Dietary Guidelines do not provide quantitative recommendations for added sugars but rather advise Americans to choose and prepare foods and beverages with little added sugars or caloric sweeteners, such as amounts suggested by the USDA's Food Guide in Appendix A-3 of the *Dietary Guidelines*. For example, Americans on a 2,000-calorie-per-day diet who divide their discretionary calorie allowance equally between solid fats and added sugars should limit consumption of added sugars to 8 teaspoons per day to comply with the *Guidelines*. According to the loss-adjusted food availability data, Americans consumed 30 teaspoons of added sugars and sweeteners per person per day in 2005. This amount suggests that Americans, on average, are consuming more than triple the amount recommended. Thirty teaspoons of added sugars and sweeteners are equivalent to 477 calories per day, or about 24 percent of the total daily caloric intake for a person on a 2,000-calorie-per-day diet.

Table 8. Per Capita Availability of Added Sugars and Sweetenersgrew 19 Percent between 1970 and 2005

Item	Per capita availability[1]		Change, 1970 to 2005	2005 loss-adjusted food availability[2]
	1970	2005		
	Pounds, dry-weight equivalent		*Percent*	*Teaspoons*
Refined cane and beet sugars	101.8	62.8	-38	13.2
Corn sweeteners	15.9	77.4	387	16.3
High-fructose corn				
syrup	.5	59.0	10,673	12.4
Glucose	10.7	15.2	43	3.2
Dextrose	4.6	3.2	-31	.7
Edible syrups	.5	.3	-32	.1
Honey	1.0	1.0	3	.2
Total sugars and				
sweeteners	119.1	141.6	19	29.8

Note: Totals may not add due to rounding.

[1] Aggregate data, unadjusted for cooking losses, plate waste, and other losses.

[2] Adjusted for cooking losses, plate waste, and other losses. One teaspoon of sugarequals 16 calories.

Source: USDA, ERS Food Availability (Per Capita) DataSystem.

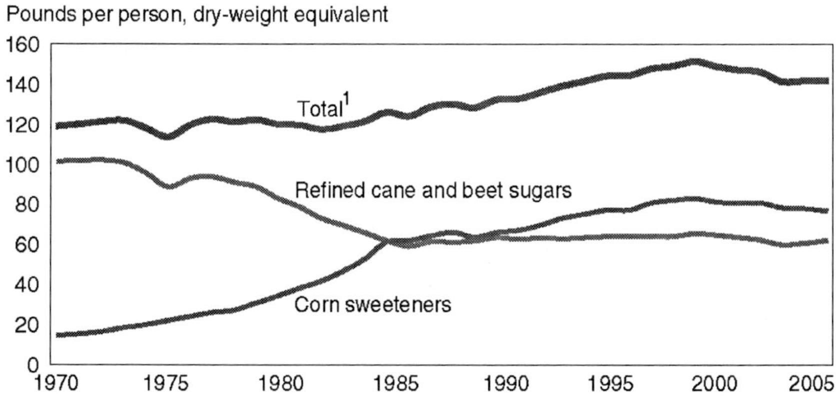

[1]Includes honey, maple, and sugarcane syrup, edible molasses, and edible refiners' syrup.

Source: USDA, ERS Food Availability (Per Capita) Data System.

Figure 7. Corn sweetener consumption increased 387 percent between 1970 and 2005.

References

American Dietetic Association. *Nutrition and You: Trends 2002: Final Report of Findings*, October 2002, www.eatright.org/ada/files/trends02 findings.pdf.

Blayney, D., Miller, J. & Stillman. R. (1995). *Dairy: Background for 1995 Farm Legislation*, AER-705, U.S. Department of Agriculture, Economic Research Service, April www.ers.usda.gov/Publications/aer705/.

Buzby, J. & Farah, H. (2006). "Chicken Consumption Continues Longrun Rise," *Amber Waves*, U.S. Department of Agriculture, Economic Research Service, *Vol. 4*, Issue 2 (April 2006) p. 5, www.ers.usda.gov/Amber Waves/April06/Findings/Chicken.htm.

Buzby, Jean C., Wells, H. F. & Vocke, G. (2006). *Possible Implication for U.S. Agriculture from Adoption of Select Dietary Guidelines*, ERR-31, U.S. Department of Agriculture, *Economic Research Service*, www.ers.usda.gov/Publications/ERR31/.

Buzby, J., Farah, H. & Vocke, G. (2005). "Will 2005 be the Year of the Whole Grain?" *Amber Waves*, U.S. Department of Agriculture, *Economic Research Service, Vol. 3,* Issue 3 (June) 2-7, www.ers.usda.gov/Amber-Waves/June05/Features/Will2005WholeGrain.htm.

Farah, H. & Buzby, J. (2005). "U.S. Food Consumption Up 16 Percent Since 1970," *Amber Waves*, *Vol. 3*, Issue 5 (November) p. 5, www.ers.usda.gov/amberwaves/november05/findings/usfoodconsumption.htm/.

Kantor, L. (1998). *A Dietary Assessment of the U.S. Food Supply: Comparing Per Capita Food Consumption with Food Guide Pyramid Serving Recommenda-tions*, AER-772, U.S. Department of Agriculture, Economic Research Service, December, www.ers.usda.gov/publications/aer772/.

Lucier, G. & Jerardo, A. (2005). *Vegetables and Melons Situation and Outlook Yearbook*, VGS, U.S. Department of Agriculture, Economic Research Service, July 2005, www.ers.usda.gov/publications/vgs/JulyYeabook 2005/VGS2005.pdf.

Moore, William. (1991). "Trends in U.S. Soft Drink Consumption—Demand Implications for Low-Calorie and Other Sweeteners," *Sugar and Sweeteners: Situation and Outlook Report*, U.S.Department of Agriculture, Economic Research Service, September.

Pollack, S. & Perez, A. (2005). *Fruit and Tree Nuts Situation and Outlook Year-book*, FTS, U.S. Department of Agriculture, Economic Research Service, October 2005, www.ers.usda.gov/publications/FTS/Yearbook05/FTS2005.pdf

Pollack, S. "Consumer Demand for Fruit and Vegetables: The U.S. Example," *Changing Structure of Global Food Consumption and Trade, Agriculture and Trade Report,* WRS-01-1, U.S. Department of Agriculture,

Economic Research Service, May (2001). 49-54, www.ers.usda.gov/publications/wrs011/wrs011.pdf/.

Putnam, J., Allshouse, J. & Kantor, L. S. (2002). "U.S. Per Capita Food Supply Trends: More Calories, Refined Carbohydrates, and Fats," *FoodReview*, *Vol, 25*, Issue 3 (December) 2-15, www.ers.usda.gov/publications/FoodReview/DEC2002/frvol25i3a.pdf

Stewart, H., Blisard, N., Bhuyan, S. & Nayga, R. (2005). Jr. *Demand for Food Away from Home: Full-Service or Fast Food?* AER-829, U.S. Department of Agriculture, Economic Research Service, www.ers.usda.gov/publications/AER829/.

U. S. Department of Agriculture. "Profiling Food Consumption in America," *Agriculture Fact Book 2001-2002*, 2003, www.usda.gov/factbook/chapter2.htm/.

U.S. Department of Agriculture. *My Pyramid.gov: Steps to a Healthier You.* April 2005, http://www.mypyramid.gov/.

U.S. Department of Agriculture, Economic Research Service. *ERS Food Availability Data*, April 2006, www.ers.usda.gov/data/foodconsumption/foodavailindex.htm/

U.S. Department of Agriculture, Economic Research Service. *ERS Loss-Adjusted Food Availability Data*, April 2006, www.ers.usda.gov/data/foodconsumption/foodguideindex.htm/

U.S. Department of Health and Human Services. *Dietary Guidelines for Americans,* January 2005, sixth edition, www.health.gov/dietaryguidelines/

U.S. Department of Health and Human Services, Centers for Disease Control and Prevention. "Americans Slightly Taller, Much Heavier Than Four Decades Ago," *Advance Data From Vital and Health Statistics, 347* (October 27, 2004).

U.S. Department of Health and Human Services, Centers for Disease Control and Prevention. "*Behavioral Risk Factor Surveillance System Prevalence Data,*" October 13, 2006, http://apps.nccd.cdc.gov/brfss/

U.S. Department of Health and Human Services, Centers for Disease Control and Prevention, National Center for Health Statistics. "Overweight" data links, February 12, 2007, www.cdc.gov/nchs/fastats/overwt.htm/

Variyam, J. & E. Golan. "New Health Information is Reshaping Food Choices," *FoodReview*, U.S. Department of Agriculture, *Economic Research Service, Vol. 25*, Issue 1 (May 2002) pp. 13-18, www.ers.usda.gov/ publications/FoodReview/May2002/frvol25i1c.pdf/

Wells, H. & J. Buzby. "ERS Food Availability Data Look at Consumption in Three Ways," *Amber Waves*, U.S. Dept. of Agriculture, *Economic Research Service, Vol. 5*, Issue 3 (June 2007) pp. 40-41, www.ers.usda.gov/ AmberWaves/june07/DataFeature/

End Notes

[1] Legumes (i.e., dry beans, peas, and lentils) count as a daily allowance in either the meat or the vegetable group. In this report, we included legumes in the vegetable group. ERS does not have data on seeds, such as pumpkin, sunflower, and squash seeds.

[2] ERS compiles data for the major manufactured fat and oil products, that is, margarine, edible tallow, lard, shortening, and salad and cooking oils. The food availability data aggregate them into an added fats and oils group and do not provide estimates of dietary fat from food sources, such as meat and dairy.

[3] See www.ers.usda.gov/Data/FoodConsumption/ for detailed documentation of the data system.

[4] Putnam et al. (2002) estimated that Americans consumed 0.6 oz-eq of whole-grains per person per day in 2000 that were not included in the loss-adjusted food availability data. Buzby et

al. (2006) estimated that 0.261 oz-eq of whole-wheat flour and whole-wheat flour products are covered in the food availability database by using the estimated per capita consumption of 5.22 oz-eq of wheat flour per person and the 5-percent industry estimate of whole-wheat flour as a share of domestically milled wheat (Buzby et al., 2006). If the missing whole-grain foods of 0.6 oz-eq wereadded to the 0.261 oz-eq already covered in the data, we estimate that the new total for whole grains would be about 0.9 oz-eq in 2005.

[5] In our analysis, only the milk portions of half and half and eggnog are included in the daily dairy amount. Cream portions of these products, cream cheese, and butter are counted as added fats.

[6] The *Guidelines* recommend that fats and oils, both naturally occurring and added, contribute 20 to 35 percent of total calories for adults; 25 to 35 percent for children 4 to 18 years old; and 30 to 35 percent for children 2 to 3 years old.

[7] Cream portions of half and half and eggnog, as well as cream cheese and butter, are counted as added fats.

[8] According to MyPyramid Plan, meat, poultry, and fish are counted in total ounces. For the other foods in this group, the following portions are counted as the equivalent of 1 ounce of cooked lean meat: 1 egg, ¼ cup of cooked dry beans, ¼ cup of tofu, a 2ounce soy burger, and 1 tablespoon of peanut butter. Legumes (i.e., dry beans, peas, and lentils) count either as a daily allowance in the meat or the vegetable group. In this report, we included legumes in the vegetable group. ERS does not have data on seeds.

CHAPTER SOURCES

The following chapters have been previously published:

Chapter 1 – This is an edited, excerpted and augmented edition of a United States Department of Agriculture, Economic Research Service, Economic Research Report Number 62, dated August 2008.

Chapter 2 – This is an edited, excerpted and augmented edition of a United States Department of Agriculture, Economic Research Service, Economic Research Report Number 43, dated June 2007.

Chapter 3 – This is an edited, excerpted and augmented edition of a United States Department of Agriculture, Economic Research Service, Economic Information Bulletin Number 33, dated March 2008.

INDEX

D

E

F

G

H

N

O

P

R

S